BIG
BOOB

BIG BOOB

a memoir

Finding Hope and Optimism
Through Inflammatory Breast Cancer

EMILY JUNGBLUT

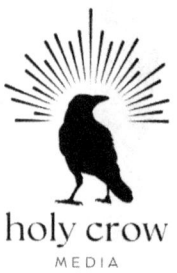

holy crow
MEDIA

© Copyright 2026
Emily Jungblut-Swinarski
All rights reserved.

This material may in no way be copied, reprinted, or shown in any medium without the express written consent of the author.

Paperback ISBN: 979-8-90183-000-0
Hardcover ISBN: 979-8-90183-001-7
eBook ISBN: 979-8-90183-002-4

Printed in the United States of America

This book is intended for informational and educational purposes only. The author is not a physician, medical professional, or healthcare provider, and the content of this book is not intended to be a substitute for professional medical advice, diagnosis, or treatment. Always seek the advice of your physician or other qualified healthcare provider.

FOR EVERY PERSON AFFECTED BY
INFLAMMATORY BREAST CANCER.
I SEE YOU. I LOVE YOU.

CONTENTS

INTRODUCTION i
CHAPTER 1 - FEELING MY BOOBIES 1
CHAPTER 2 - STOP FREAKING OUT 3
CHAPTER 3 - WAIT AND SEE 7
CHAPTER 4 - CAT SCAN 13
CHAPTER 5 - IMAGING DAY 17
CHAPTER 6 - THE CALL 27
CHAPTER 7 - SHARING THE NEWS 31
CHAPTER 8 - CALM BEFORE THE STORM 37
CHAPTER 9 - NOT FROM THIS 41
CHAPTER 10 - BLANKETS 47
CHAPTER 11 - I DID EVERYTHING RIGHT 51
CHAPTER 12 - A RARITY 55
CHAPTER 13 - SCANXIETY 61
CHAPTER 14 - SATURDAY MORNING 63
CHAPTER 15 - MAKING A PLAN 65
CHAPTER 16 - SKINNY NECK 71
CHAPTER 17 - FIRST CHEMO 75
CHAPTER 18 - HE HELD ME 83
CHAPTER 19 - SHAVING MY HEAD 89
CHAPTER 20 - RAINBOW CHARTS 93
CHAPTER 21 - PORT FAIL 97
CHAPTER 22 - MOM COMES TO TOWN 101
CHAPTER 23 - LIKE A HOLE IN MY CHEST 105
CHAPTER 24 - DOVE AND OTHER JOYS 109
CHAPTER 25 - A NEW HOBBY 115
CHAPTER 26 - CIRCLES OF SUPPORT 117

CHAPTER 27 - WIG 121
CHAPTER 28 - THERAPY CAT 125
CHAPTER 29 - NOT DOING THIS ANYMORE 129
CHAPTER 30 - THE SMILING STRANGER EFFECT 133
CHAPTER 31 - THE TOLL OF STRESS 137
CHAPTER 32 - THE IN-LAWS ARE COMING 141
CHAPTER 33 - BOOBS FOR SCIENCE 143
CHAPTER 34 - A LETTER TO MY BOOBS 145
CHAPTER 35 - FEELING THEM FOR THE LAST TIME ... 147
CHAPTER 36 - I'M FLAT NOW 151
CHAPTER 37 - TWO OF EVERYTHING 155
CHAPTER 38 - FIRST LOOK 159
CHAPTER 39 - CANCER-FREE 161
CHAPTER 40 - PEOPLE SAY WEIRD THINGS 165
CHAPTER 41 - PEOPLE SAY SUPPORTIVE THINGS 177
CHAPTER 42 - SNAKE UNDER MY SKIN 181
CHAPTER 43 - THE IN-LAWS ARE LEAVING 185
CHAPTER 44 - MORE CHEMO 187
CHAPTER 45 - RADIATION 191
CHAPTER 46 - BURNT TO A CRISP 197
CHAPTER 47 - A NINETIES SITCOM 203
CHAPTER 48 - REAL-LIFE ANGELS 207
CHAPTER 49 - WEDDING 209
CHAPTER 50 - THE REVOLVING DOOR AND
RELATIONSHIPS 213
CHAPTER 51 - MY "OLD SELF" 217
CHAPTER 52 - THE END? 223
HELPFUL RECIPES 227
GRATITUDE 229
BIBLIOGRAPHY 233
ABOUT THE AUTHOR 235

INTRODUCTION

WHEN I WAS DIAGNOSED with inflammatory breast cancer (IBC) at age thirty-five, I was desperate for stories of hope and survival.

IBC is the most aggressive and deadly form of breast cancer, and the statistics were terrifying. The reported five-year survival rate was just 39 percent when I was diagnosed, according to the American Cancer Society. I searched for hopeful content and a promise that I'd make it to the other side. I clung to the few stories I could find from those still living.

When I was going through chemotherapy, unsure of my future and feeling like a pile of smashed trash, I vowed that if I survived this cancer, I would share hope and optimism with others. I wanted to be the survival story I so desperately sought in my darkest days.

Writing this in the years following my journey was highly therapeutic. While I intended to write this book for those seeking hope and wanting to know about the nitty-gritty of IBC, I may have also written it for myself. For the me who needed to process the heaviness. For the me who needed a laugh at how bizarre it all was. And for the past me who needed the present me to tell her that everything would be OK.

The stories and experiences I write about are just that—my experiences. While every detail might not be completely accurate because chemo brain and brain fog are real, I write about my experiences as I remember them happening. In addition, some names and minor details have been changed to protect the identities of health-care workers and those who must remain anonymous. You know, for legal reasons.

I feel I should give a trigger warning for cancer (obviously), suicidal thoughts, and the topics of death and death planning. I use swear words. I talk about poop. I find humor in uncomfortable situations. I get personal because I don't want to sugarcoat how cruel, difficult, and weird cancer treatment is. Sometimes it's even funny.

My experience is that of stage IIIC inflammatory breast cancer. While all IBC cases are either stage III or IV, these stages, their treatment protocols, and the realities of each patient can be vastly different. I was not diagnosed with stage IV, also called metastatic cancer, and I acknowledge that the experiences of those with stage IV IBC are different from those with stage III. While I write about fear of death and scary statistics, it is never my intention to offend or minimize the experiences of other patients with a terminal prognosis. I am simply sharing my own thoughts and feelings about navigating IBC and everything it brings with it.

Here's some information about IBC and statistics from the time of my diagnosis, just so we all know what we're going into.

According to the National Cancer Institute's website, "Inflammatory breast cancer is a rare and very aggressive disease in which cancer cells block lymph vessels in the skin of the breast."

According to the American Cancer Society, IBC accounts for 1 to 5 percent of all breast cancers diagnosed in the United States. It causes symptoms of breast inflammation like swelling and redness. All inflammatory breast cancers start at stage III since they involve the skin. The five-year survival rate for all stages of IBC is 39 percent for women diagnosed between 2012 and 2018. I was diagnosed in 2021, but survival statistics for this period have not been made available at the time of writing this book.

This is my official disclaimer that I am not a doctor or medical professional of any kind. As an IBC survivor, I am providing my own experiences for educational and entertainment purposes only. The content in this book should not be taken as medical advice. Before making any decisions about your own health, please consult your health-care provider.

CHAPTER 1
FEELING MY BOOBIES

THE NEW YEAR was off to a great start. The decorations were put away, and I began my annual household decluttering project. I found it refreshing and therapeutic to go through each room and donate what no longer served me. There was even talk of a COVID-19 vaccine being made available in the coming months. I was hopeful that we would soon rejoin society and start living our lives again.

A week into January, I was feeling my boobies in the shower just as I did every day. Arms crossed, left hand holding the right boob, right hand holding the left. As the water flowed over my back, I was thrown out of my boobie-holding meditation. My left boob could no longer fit into my hand. One hand felt like it was holding an apple, and the other felt like it was holding a cantaloupe.

This doesn't seem right, I thought. I knew I had gained a few pounds during the global pandemic. After all, the entire world was in survival mode, and I assumed everyone had gained some extra weight. That's also what happens when you spend a full year perfecting banana bread and the world's best cheesy chicken recipe—not to be eaten together, unless you like that kind of thing.

The fluttery sensation of anxiety filled my stomach. I became short of breath. The water suddenly felt colder. I knew in my gut that something wasn't right. This was not normal.

I knew my boobs. I *really* knew them. I'd felt my boobies every day for the last 5,400 days, give or take a few. I knew every fiber of breast tissue, every skin imperfection, and every rogue hair that I'd occasionally pluck.

I decided to give myself an actual breast exam right there in the shower—an exam like the ones you see in the pamphlets at the gynecologist's office.

Apart from feeling my own boobs, I received annual breast exams at the doctor's office. I knew how it went. I knew the motions—fingers moving up and down, assessing the breast like a grid. First up, then down, then in a spiral motion.

Not only was my left boob significantly bigger than the other, but it had also grown denser. It wasn't as bouncy or squishy as the right side. It felt heavy and firm.

As my fingers spiraled around in a circle, I came to the lower, inner area of my breast, just outside the nipple. It wasn't easy to feel. Because the tissue was so thick, I felt the need to dig deep. It felt even more dense than the rest.

Is this a lump? I asked myself. This was not what I imagined a lump would feel like. I imagined a squishy boob with a hard marble-sized round thing. In my head, *that's* what a lump was. Not this. This wasn't the marble within a squish. This was a big hard boob. Something was very, very wrong.

My heart rate sped up, and my breath quickened as adrenaline filled my body.

Shit, I thought. *I think I have cancer.*

CHAPTER 2

STOP FREAKING OUT

"OH MY GOD! Oh my God! Oh my God!"

I couldn't stop saying it. A knot formed in my throat, and I felt like vomiting. How could this be real? How could something bad be happening? I was only thirty-five years old. I was young. This didn't happen to women in their thirties.

I jumped out of the shower and ran into the bedroom, still dripping wet with boobies and bits on full display.

"Jonathan!" I screamed. "Come here!"

My husband of thirteen years walked down the hallway holding his coffee mug in his usual nonchalant way.

"I think I found a lump!" I yelled in his face. "I found a lump. Feel this, feel this!" I was in the midst of a severe freakout, hyperventilating and yelling at 700 words per minute about lumps and boobs as I stood there naked in our bedroom.

He put his mug down on my dresser. "Slow down and breathe," he said. "What happened?"

"I felt my boobs in the shower, and there's a spot." I grabbed his hand and placed it on my boob in the exact place where I had felt it. "Feel right here. Can you feel it?"

"Stop freaking out. It's probably nothing." Jonathan was the calm one in our marriage. I was more high-strung and prone to the occasional breakdown over the small stuff.

"Why would you say it's nothing? It's something. I know it is."

I made him push on my boob again to feel the dense area on the inner side of my left nipple. While he was pushing and examining, I tried to calm down, but I was crying so hard I could barely find my words.

"I see what you mean. But I don't think it feels like a lump."

"Well, what the hell is it then, huh? This isn't normal." I was defensive. I was confused. I was scared.

"If you're concerned about it, just send a message to the doctor." There. Problem solved. Cool, calm, collected. Jonathan was a fixer. No matter the crisis, his mind always went to the quickest solution.

"But what if it's nothing?" My preconceived notion of what a lump was supposed to be had me second-guessing what I was feeling.

"You'll be worried about it until you know for sure." He knew me well. I *would* be hysterical until I knew what it was.

My body had air-dried by this point, so I got dressed. I called the health clinic. Even if I was making a huge issue out of nothing, I wasn't going to wait.

A woman answered the appointment line. Her voice sounded warm and calm, exactly what my nerves needed. I told her what happened in the shower and asked if I could get an appointment with my primary care provider as soon as possible.

"The earliest I have is next week."

This was only Monday. *Next week?* I thought. *That's not soon enough.* But I took it.

I hung up and stood in my room, pacing in a tight circle with my right hand cupping my boob. There was no way I was going to wait until next week. Swaying and pacing, I brainstormed how to find a loophole to surpass the system.

As the firstborn child, I was a natural rule follower. I accepted what I was told and was eager to please my parents and the adults around me. After all, didn't grown-ups know best? But I was the grown-up now. The older I got, the more willing I became to ask for forgiveness rather than permission. In serious situations, I had no problem going straight to the top.

I called the main number of the Huntsman Cancer Institute in Salt Lake City. I remembered seeing advertisements and commercials for the institute, and it looked reputable. Maybe someone would validate my worry and have advice on how to get this ball rolling faster.

It turned out they couldn't get me an appointment. But they did recommend that I have diagnostic imaging done as soon as possible. A recommendation was what I needed to be taken seriously, and I was going to use it to my advantage.

I sent a message to my PCP through the health-care app. I told the doctor that Huntsman themselves suggested I have diagnostic imaging done. *And if Huntsman says so, then it needs to be done, right?* I thought to myself. *Who could say no to that? The cancer experts themselves said I needed this.*

The PCP's nurse messaged me back within minutes, saying she had a cancellation. She asked if I could be there in two hours.

"I will be there in two hours."

CHAPTER 3

WAIT AND SEE

I SHOWED UP at the health clinic, checked in, and anxiously waited for my name to be called.

It was a cold January morning, and I was bundled up in my sweater and winter coat. I had a mask on because there were still serious concerns about contracting COVID-19. The vaccine was available only for health-care workers and high-risk cases. Breathing while anxious and worried wasn't so easy while wearing a mask. I was becoming increasingly warm and started feeling lightheaded. I thought I might pass out right there in the waiting area.

"Emily?" someone called out from the doorway. I gathered my things. As usual, I had a water bottle with me. You never know when you might spontaneously choke on your own spit and need a drink. Maybe that was something only I worried about. I tended to plan for worst-case scenarios.

In the exam room, I felt more nervous than a long-tailed cat in a room full of rocking chairs. I had only met my doctor once before, but she seemed nice enough.

"What brings you in today?" the nurse asked.

I told her everything from feeling my boobies in the shower, to Jonathan validating that he felt something weird too, to Huntsman's imaging suggestion. I was desperate to be taken seriously. A woman I knew through the military spouse community had faced more than a year of her doctor brushing off her concerns, only to find out she had stage III breast cancer after getting a second opinion. I didn't want that to be me. I gave every detail I could possibly think of. Anything to prevent being brushed off.

The nurse left the room to get the doctor. A few minutes later, she walked in.

The vibe was off. Way off. You know that feeling when someone has already made up their mind before even talking to you? This was that. I instantly knew my concerns were about to be dismissed, and I was terrified. I felt my defensive guard rise.

Before examining me, she mentioned how unlikely it was that anything was wrong for so many reasons. I was too young. I didn't have a family history of breast cancer. I was premenopausal, so a swollen breast was likely hormonal.

"I know my body," I said after listening to her explain my symptoms away without even a simple examination. "I've had a period for twenty-four years, and nothing hormonal has ever caused anything like this before. This isn't normal. Something is wrong."

"Would you like me to do a physical exam?" she asked.

"Yes!" I replied. Of course I wanted a physical exam. Wasn't that what I was there for? I was there because I was convinced I had a tumor. *Please feel my boobs, lady.*

I didn't wait for her to leave the room to undress. I whipped off my shirt in her full view, boobies out with no time to waste. Topless, I didn't hide my bra under my shirt or neatly fold it on the chair. I gave zero fucks about modesty. I just wanted to know what was wrong with me.

"Do you see how they're different sizes?" I asked in a frenzied voice, pointing back and forth between my boobs. My cheeks flushed out of sheer desperation to be heard.

"Not really," she said dismissively. "Lie back on the table, and I'll do an exam."

I lay back as she pressed on each of my boobs in a patterned motion, just as I had done in the shower. Just like the pamphlets showed how to do it. Up and down and back up again. Around in a circle. Then she squeezed my nipple.

"Holy shit," I said, caught by surprise. That had never happened during any routine breast exam I'd ever had. She squeezed harder and harder as if trying to pop a zit. It hurt, and I winced in pain.

"Well, I said it would be uncomfortable. And no discharge is coming out."

"No, I don't have discharge," I replied. I had never said I did. "There's a dense spot right here." I pointed to the precise location on the outside edge of my nipple.

She pressed lightly around that area, barely a quarter of an inch into the tissue. "I don't feel anything concerning. Sit up and let's talk about it."

I sat up on the table, put my bra and shirt back on, and moved to a regular chair.

"Well, I'm not appreciating a mass in your breast," she said. *I'm not appreciating it either*, I thought. I then realized that wasn't what she meant. She meant she didn't feel what I was feeling. "Of course, I'm not in your body, I'm only feeling it from the outside. But I don't feel anything concerning."

I felt like a full-blown hypochondriac. Was I making this up? Was there even a dense spot? Was I being paranoid, creating something out of nothing? But I knew I wasn't. And I wasn't going to let her gaslight me into thinking I'd gone bananas.

"Can't you at least see that one boob is bigger than the other?" I asked, desperate for any sliver of validation.

"I can see it's not exactly the same as the other," she answered. "That can be normal, though. Especially since you're premenopausal. It could be hormonal changes, like I said. I think we should wait six months and see what happens."

Wait six months and see what happens? Are you freaking kidding me?

There was no way I was going to wait six months, full of fear every day that I might have cancer. The thought of what could happen in six months horrified me.

"No," I said firmly. "No. I'm not going to wait and see. I want to have a mammogram." It was the first time I had ever said no to a doctor. It felt rebellious. I felt slightly rude, like one of those people who tells someone else how to do their job.

"I really think it's hormonal," she said with conviction, pushing back at my rebellion. "It's so unlikely that anything will show up on a mammogram. Mammograms usually don't show anything in young, denser breasts anyway."

"I understand that." I sat up straighter, gathering any thread of gumption I could. I doubled down. "But I *know* my body. And something is wrong. I want a mammogram."

My insides started vibrating, like I was about to burst into tears at any moment. Pushing back like this felt incredibly unnatural. I wasn't a rebel, but when your intuition knows, it knows. I felt in my guts like this could be my life on the line, and I wasn't going to take no for an answer. This choice to firmly say no, and mean it, was the best decision I could have made.

"I'll tell you what," she said, about to give in. "I'll order an ultrasound."

"OK," I replied. It was better than nothing.

The only thing I knew for sure was that I was *not* going to be waiting and seeing.

CHAPTER 4
CAT SCAN

THE WAITING PERIOD between that initial appointment and imaging day was brutal. A sour, acidic worry filled my throat without ceasing.

I made the strategic decision to keep what was happening to myself. I didn't tell anyone—not my mom, not my sister, not my best friends. The only ones who knew were Jonathan and me. I didn't want to worry anyone if it turned out to be a whole bunch of nothing, if I was, in fact, a giant hypochondriac. My mom is a natural worrier, like most mothers, and I didn't want to be the cause of additional stress. I pretended like everything was normal.

My ultrasound appointment wasn't until Friday the following week—more than ten days away.

"I feel like I'm going to implode from stress," I told Jonathan one night as we were watching television.

"One day at a time," he reminded me. "We don't know for sure until we know for sure."

It was becoming clear to both of us that something bad was happening inside my body. The pain got worse, and my boob felt harder, bigger, and more inflamed by the day. My mind couldn't focus on anything other than what was going on with my boob. I had boobs on the brain constantly. I spent most of my time sitting on the living room couch in a foggy daze. I tried reading to pass the time, but retaining words was beyond my ability. I found myself rereading every other paragraph, forgetting what I had just taken in.

I would have given anything to get out of the house, to meet up with a friend for lunch, anything to keep my mind distracted. But I didn't have many friends in Utah. Not yet anyway.

After thirteen years of active-duty military service, Jonathan received an opportunity to work at an Air National Guard unit in Salt Lake City. I grew up on the East Coast, so Utah might just as well have been Mars. I didn't know much about it, and I didn't know anyone who lived there. But taking the job in Salt Lake City would mean we would no longer have to move every two to three years. And he probably wouldn't deploy again, or at least not nearly as often. That sounded like heaven to me, putting down roots and making a "forever home."

"Sign us up," I told him. So he did.

We moved to Utah in September 2019. I spent a few months unpacking, getting the house organized, and learning the ropes of living in a new town. A few months later, I was finally feeling ready to get out, make friends, and be part of the community. Then the world shut down and turned inward. A global pandemic was not what I expected for 2020, but there we were, in a new state, far from family and friends, on our own. We made the best of it, though, using the time to be productive. We repainted the entire interior of our home, ceilings included. I set up my new Reiki business, excited to follow my own ambitions, as my dreams had taken a back seat while supporting Jonathan's military career.

But now I desperately needed a friend's company to keep me distracted from boobie hell. Other than Jonathan, the only friends around were my cats.

Bradley and Felix were more like my children than pets. Maybe every childless pet parent says that, but it feels true. I hadn't worked outside the home for more than ten years, thanks to military life, and most of my time was spent in their company. They were my babies, and I was their mother.

No matter where I went, it felt like one of them was always with me, a little black shadow constantly on my trail. With short black hair and copperish-green eyes, they each had a doglike personality. They played fetch and liked going outside on a leash to play in the snow or chase bugs.

When we were inside, if I was sitting, one of them was sure to be on my lap or resting next to me, sleeping, bathing, or purring to his heart's content. And when I was in a daze on the couch, blankly staring at the TV screen, they were there.

Each of them took turns lying on my lap and keeping me company. They could sense that my mental state was unwell. Animals seem to know these things, giving extra cuddles when you're feeling low. I wasn't prepared for the bizarreness of what happened next.

Independent of each other, without the other witnessing it, both cats began touching my left boob, my big boob, as they lay on me—paw outstretched to touch my breast.

I had heard that animals could sense cancer in humans. Was that what they were doing? Did they know something I didn't know yet?

According to the Cancer Council of Australia, several studies have shown that animals may detect differences in body odors between healthy people and cancer patients, especially for lung, breast, and prostate cancers.

Did I smell like cancer? Was I losing my mind? My logical brain had clearly leaped out the window if I thought my cats could smell cancer. But maybe they could.

"Look at this," I said to Jonathan the first time Felix outstretched his paw to my boob. "He's touching my left boob. I think he's giving me a cat scan. Hahaha." If my mind had left me, at least my humor was still intact.

"Aww, he knows you don't feel good," he said. He picked up his phone and took a picture.

CHAPTER 5
IMAGING DAY

THE NEXT FRIDAY finally rolled around, and the weight on my chest, both literally and figuratively, was unbearable. The mental Tilt-A-Whirl my mind had been riding was gearing up for its final spin.

Jonathan was off work every Friday, one of the perks of his new job. I was glad he could accompany me to my appointment. When we walked in, we were the two youngest people in the waiting area. I shouldn't have been surprised. Most people our age were probably at work, taking their kids to school, living their lives, not in a radiology clinic for cancer screening.

"Hi, I'm Emily. I'm here for my ultrasound," I said in a quiet voice out of fear that if I spoke those words louder, the universe would be granted permission to inflict more damage.

The woman behind the check-in desk scrunched her eyebrows as she studied her computer screen. "It looks like you're going to have a mammogram."

"Oh?" I said. "I thought it was an ultrasound."

"It was, but that's not our protocol. We do a diagnostic mammogram first, and if anything shows up abnormal, we'll do an ultrasound. But a mammogram comes first."

Great, I thought. *Mammograms are meant to pick up problems with boobs. This is exactly what I need.*

A mammographer walked around the corner and called my name. Jonathan had to stay in the waiting room due to the COVID-19 protocol. I gave him a kiss and followed her to the back.

"I'm Sarah, and I'll be helping you today." She guided me to a changing room. "Just change into this gown, then wait on the couch right there."

I was sitting on the couch for less than a minute when she came back.

"You're only thirty-five years old?" she asked. "What brings you in for a mammogram? Women usually don't get them until they're forty."

I dropped the gown to my waist and showed her my boobs. I'd normally feel self-conscious about taking my clothes off to show a stranger my naked body, but at this point, I'd strip in front of anyone if I thought they could help me. Modesty was officially out the window.

"Do you see how they're different?" I said, trying to keep my fervor under wraps. "And the left one is getting bigger and harder and starting to hurt badly. I think my nipple might be starting to invert, too."

The pain amped up the day after the first doctor squeezed it like a zit. But my boob wasn't a zit. It was a boob. And it didn't pop. It just hurt worse and worse.

"Oh yes. I see what you're talking about."

"You do?" I was relieved. "You see that they're different sizes, and the left one is hard?" I was still begging for someone to validate what I was seeing and feeling, someone to confirm that I wasn't making it all up.

In the mammography room, Sarah showed me how to stand as she placed my boobs to be squished by the machine. My left boob was imaged first, and I'd never known greater pain. It was already hard and aching, and having it smooshed and pressed was torture. Thankfully, Sarah was good at her job, so the smooshing and squishing were over quickly.

After the agony of the left side, it was my right boob's turn. It wasn't as excruciating as the left and felt more uncomfortable than anything else. Easy-peasy in comparison.

The mammogram was over, and I returned to the couch in the patient waiting area. I was the only person in the room and was still separated from Jonathan. I hated not being able to tell him how it was going. I hated not being able to tell him how scary this was, how I was sure my boob was going to pop in that machine. But I couldn't. So I waited, wondering if he was worrying about me too.

Sarah opened the door a few minutes later and came inside. "It looks like nothing obvious showed up on the mammogram. But the doctor wants to go ahead and do an ultrasound."

"If nothing showed up, why does he want to do an ultrasound?" I asked, remembering what the lady at the check-in desk had said about their protocol.

"Because it looks like there may be a slight thickening to the skin, so we just want to make sure it's nothing serious." Even though her voice was calm and eased my worry, I knew this couldn't be good. "The ultrasound is better at detecting problems in dense breasts like yours."

I wasn't sure if I should be relieved or afraid. For a moment, I felt relieved. Nothing was found on the mammogram. It didn't show any tumors or cysts or anything obvious. That part was great news. But the skin looked thick. And that didn't sound like great news.

Sarah led me to a young doctor who was waiting. He introduced himself as Brian, an imaging resident. He made me feel comfortable with small talk as I lay down on the table.

"How's your morning going?"

Well, I'm here getting scanned for cancer, Brian. Not so great.

"Are you from here?"

My Philadelphia accent probably gave away that I'm not.

"This will be so easy. Not nearly as difficult as the mammogram."

This is great news, Brian. I can't handle that again.

He had me lift my left arm so he could better access the area he'd be looking at. "What do you like to do for fun?" he asked.

With my brain feeling like mush, the only thing I could think of to say was "hiking."

Brian squeezed the jelly onto my boob and used the ultrasound scanner to look at what was going on. As he moved the device around and pressed buttons, I asked why he decided to do an ultrasound if the mammogram was clear.

"Sarah said your breast looked abnormal, and mammograms can sometimes miss things in young women with denser breasts. So we just want to make sure nothing is hiding deeper in the tissue." I wanted to jump off the table in joy. Someone else was finally validating that I wasn't a wacko. My boob really *did* look abnormal.

I tilted my head to get a good look at the screen, curious about what it looked like. I accompanied a friend to a pregnancy ultrasound once and had picked up on a thing or two. I had no medical background and certainly wasn't an expert, but I'm a smart person. I thought maybe I would notice if something looked wonky.

Everything was going smoothly until he paused on a black circle. Still in a conversation about what hiking paths we liked to visit, he pressed button after button. It seemed like he was taking measurements of the black circle. The scanning device, which I later learned is called a transducer, was over the exact area on the edge of my nipple where it was densest, the area my PCP didn't appreciate.

"What's that?" I asked, taking a sharp turn in conversation.

Hiking? Never heard of it. I'm a big fan of black circles right now. Tell me all about them, Brian.

I was aware that medical professionals usually don't tell you what they're seeing while the scan is still happening. You typically have to wait until the report is written and reviewed by the attending physician. But Brian was friendly and nice, so I figured it couldn't hurt to ask. The worst he could say was that he couldn't talk about it.

"This looks like a potential cyst or tumor," he said.

Potential. Sounds noncommittal. You know, allegedly. For legal reasons. I understood he couldn't give me definite answers, but I wanted to know more about this "potential."

He pointed out a white border around the black circle. "This looks like a calcium layer, which is pretty typical in cancerous tumors."

Pretty typical in cancerous tumors? Did Brian just tell me that I have cancer? My jaw slowly opened, and my heart skipped a beat.

"Let me take a look at your armpit if you don't mind." I wasn't sure what my armpit had to do with anything, but OK. He squeezed more jelly into my left armpit and reached farther across my chest to scan. "I'm just taking a look at your lymph nodes." He was pushing buttons and taking measurements again.

"Are my lymph nodes bad?" I asked. I didn't know much about lymph nodes.

"This one here is five millimeters," he said, still doing his thing. "We like to see nodes smaller than four millimeters, so I'm just taking note of it." I was surprised by how much information he was sharing in the moment.

A few more moves around my pit and clicks on the keyboard, and we were done. As Brian finished up, he gave me a towel to wipe the jelly from my chest.

"Is anyone here with you? Anyone in the waiting room?"

"My husband, Jonathan, is in the main waiting room."

"Is it OK if I bring him back here?" he asked. I agreed. I needed the comfort of Jonathan's presence after what just happened.

I changed back into my clothes and could hear Brian and Jonathan chatting in the hallway. When I came out of the changing room, they were both standing there waiting for me.

"You doing OK?" Brian asked.

"I think so," I said.

"I'm hoping it's nothing to be worried about, but can you come back at one o'clock? I want to do a biopsy today."

Today? A biopsy today? I had heard of people waiting weeks to get a biopsy, and he wanted me to come back today? Despite the friendly tone of his voice, this sounded serious.

"Yeah," I nodded in agreement. "We can come back at one."

Jonathan and I left the clinic and sat in the parking lot, both speechless. It was probably only a minute, but the stunned silence seemed to last an hour.

"What do we do?" I asked quietly. "I'm really scared."

"I think we should call my mom. Is that OK?" My mother-in-law, Karen, was a physician assistant and nurse practitioner with thirty years of medical experience.

"Yeah, that's OK. I think it's time we told some people what's going on." Jonathan picked up his phone and called his mom in New York. He explained everything that had happened over the last few weeks.

"Why didn't you tell me?" She sounded offended that we hadn't told her about any of this sooner.

"I didn't want to worry anyone in case it turned out to be nothing," I said. "But now it seems like it might be something." I don't remember what she said after that. Everything was blank.

We wondered how to pass the time. We had three hours until we had to be back. Our home was only a few minutes away, so we decided to have some lunch. I couldn't eat much and started stress cleaning instead, expending energy to keep my mind from spiraling out of control.

At one o'clock, we checked in at the radiology desk for the second time that day. Sarah came out to take me back to the same room where Brian had done my ultrasound. Jonathan stayed in the front waiting room.

Brian had a serious look on his face this time. There was no small talk or chatty nature. A middle-aged doctor, the attending physician, was also preparing instruments and equipment. He smiled at me and gave a quick nod and a "hi."

"You can take off your shirt and bra and lie down on the table when you're ready," Sarah said as she moved to the side where the monitor was. "This is going to be an ultrasound-guided core needle biopsy."

"What's a core needle biopsy?" I asked. I had never had a biopsy like this before. The only type of biopsy I was familiar with was having a mole scraped from my skin at the dermatologist's office.

"They'll numb the area and insert a hollowed-out needle into the mass," she explained. "Then they'll punch out a few cells to look at under the microscope. They'll be able to tell exactly what those cells are made of, whether it's a cyst or something else. It's a pretty big needle, but you'll be numb, so you shouldn't feel it."

My eyes locked with hers in fear. I couldn't look away.

"And I can hold your hand if you'd like."

"Yes, please," I replied. The somber tone of the room sank deeper into my body.

Sarah sat on my right, holding my hand, while Brian sat on my left, masked and gloved. He sterilized my chest and got to work quickly. The other physician stood over his shoulder, giving instructions and guidance. "Try a slightly different angle. Yes, right there."

I'm sure I squeezed Sarah's hand so hard I bruised it, but she didn't complain. If I couldn't have Jonathan there to hold my hand, I was glad to have someone kind supporting me through this. I looked at Sarah as she talked about hiking, cats, and restaurants to distract me from the sharp dagger digging around my breast. Brian must have told her I liked hiking.

Brian and the other doctor took five biopsies, three from my left breast and two from the five-millimeter axillary lymph node in my armpit.

As Sarah and the physician began cleaning up and preparing samples to send to pathology, I put my top back on and shoved the bra into my purse. There was no way I wanted to put a bra on after that poking, sticking, and stabbing. The ladies would be free for the rest of the day.

"Is it OK if I go see your husband in the waiting room?" Brian asked.

"Yeah, that's fine."

"We should know the results in a few days," he told us. "I hope by Monday."

I hoped so, too. Answers were on their way, but it was going to be a long weekend full of worry.

CHAPTER 6
THE CALL

MY HOUSE HAD never been cleaner. I spent the weekend stress cleaning, reading books I wouldn't remember, watching TV—doing anything to distract me from worry and dread.

Jonathan was stoic and appeared to be holding it together from the outside. I was a sobbing mess. Cutting vegetables made me cry. The cold wind on my face made me cry. Music made me cry. The feel of the cats' soft fur made me cry. Everything made me cry. The only thing on my mind was the possibility of having cancer, dying young, and leaving behind everyone I loved.

I kept my phone on the loudest, most obnoxious ringtone I could find. I didn't want to miss any calls. Every time my phone rang, I answered, whether I recognized the number or not. I was a telemarketer's dream.

Monday came and went without any news. Tuesday came, and the afternoon soon turned into evening. I prepared to go through another sleepless night without knowing.

Jonathan and I were sitting on the couch, thinking about what to make for dinner, when the phone jolted us from our seats. I answered as quickly as my trembling fingers could push the button.

"Hello, I'd like to speak to Emily," said the voice on the other end.

"This is Emily." I switched the call to speaker so Jonathan could hear. He sat on the coffee table across from me, his hand on my knee.

"Emily, this is the nurse from the University of Utah radiology department. I'm calling because we have the results from your biopsy."

"OK." I braced myself for the worst.

"Unfortunately, it's cancer."

With those words, everything halted and sped up at the same time. Everything felt over, yet my mind flooded with thoughts, all of them of loss and death. I clutched the phone, and Jonathan clutched my hand. I had so many questions but wasn't sure what they were. I wanted to know everything but didn't know what to ask.

"Oh," I eventually got out. "What stage is it?" It was the only thing about cancer that I could remember. Cancer was categorized in stages. The higher the number, the worse it was.

"We won't know the stage until after the oncologist sees you. There's a lot that goes into staging, but I do have some other information about your cancer if you'd like me to tell you."

My cancer. I have cancer. This is my cancer. I'm thirty-five. We don't have kids yet. We just settled down in our forever home, and she just said, "YOUR cancer."

My mind wasn't prepared for the complicated medical terms that followed. Jonathan grabbed a notebook and pen and handed it to me, knowing we both weren't going to remember anything she was about to tell us without taking notes.

"The pathologist was able to glean a good bit of information from the biopsy. Both the tumor and the lymph node are cancerous. It's something called invasive ductal carcinoma, and both areas of cancer are hormone receptor-positive."

"What does that mean?" I asked. "Hormone receptor-positive?"

"It means the cancer has receptors on it that are attracted to your hormones. Yours are attracted to both estrogen and progesterone. Think of it like the cancer is feeding on the hormones."

"That doesn't sound very good."

"Well, the good news is that this type of cancer typically responds well to treatment."

This is good news, I thought. *Maybe it's an early stage, I can get some treatment, maybe just surgery, and be done with it.* My mind tried to make sense of something I knew nothing about.

"There's a little more," she continued. "They classified it as grade two, which means it's not slow-growing, but it's not fast-growing. It's somewhere in the middle. And it's HER2-positive."

"What's HER2?" I asked. "That sounds bad, too." Every word she said made it sound worse and worse.

"It's a type of protein that has human epidermal growth factor receptors. It helps cancerous cells grow more quickly."

Human what growth what now? I was thankful for that notebook as I scribbled everything down.

"So is *this* good or bad?" I had never heard of any of these terms before. I thought cancer was cancer. I didn't know there were so many different types besides where it was in the body.

"Well, it used to be kind of a bad thing. But there have been a lot of new drugs that have come out recently to treat it, so it's not as bad as it used to be."

Not as bad as it used to be.

She finished telling me all she could, and I hung up. I sat on the edge of the couch and looked up at Jonathan. He had a solemn look on his face and reached forward to touch my shoulder.

With his touch, I lost it. My face fell into my hands, and I sobbed. I was trembling yet felt numb. All I could do was cry. Jonathan knelt on the floor at my knees and wrapped his arms around me.

"What am I going to do?" I said it over and over.

"We're going to fight this. And we're going to do it together."

CHAPTER 7
SHARING THE NEWS

EXACTLY ONE BREAKDOWN later, it was time to call my parents.

My mom and dad, Dawn and Mark, knew almost nothing about the situation. Within the last decade, they had dealt with several life-threatening situations regarding their children. I didn't tell them much because I didn't want to be the cause of any more restless nights. I had told my mom that I was having my boob looked at but tried not to make it a big deal. I made it seem like a "just in case, but it'll be fine" kind of thing.

My family lived more than two thousand miles away from where we lived in Utah. I grew up in Pennsylvania, where my parents and sister, Laura, still lived. My brother, Jeffrey, had joined the military following high school and was living in Maryland. We were all geographically separated, but we spoke often.

"Do you want to get your thoughts together before calling them?" Jonathan asked. "Maybe you should take some notes and call Jeffrey first. Like a test run before you tell your mom."

This was a good idea. If I told my brother before calling Mom, I could practice saying the words. Maybe I wouldn't cry as much when telling my parents. And if I didn't cry as much, they wouldn't be too worried. I realize now how illogical that was. Of course they would worry.

I decided to text my brother first. *Jeffrey, call me as soon as you can. It's an emergency.* He video called me right away. I could see he was at home, alone in his basement office.

"Jeffrey." As soon as I spoke, the tears started flowing uncontrollably down my face.

"Em? What's wrong, Em?" I was blubbering, my nose filling with snot as I stuttered and gasped to catch my breath mid-cry. "Is Jonathan OK?" I was sure he could think of very few scenarios that would cause such a guttural reaction within me, and someone being hurt or worse was certainly at the top of that list.

"Yeah, Jonathan's fine. He's right here." I pointed my phone's camera toward him. "But I have something really important to tell you."

"What's going on?" he asked, a concerned look overtaking his face.

"I have cancer." I barely got the words out and started to wail.

I didn't hold myself together as much as I thought I could. Telling my brother the news had only made me even more inconsolable. Seeing the deep concern on his face didn't help. Being the younger sibling, he never worried about me. I was always the one looking out for him.

As I mentally prepared to call my parents, I knew I was going to break down. I told myself that it was OK to break down. It was OK to cry. It was OK to show emotion when telling my friends and family I had cancer. It was OK to crumble. It was OK to be vulnerable, especially with the people who loved me most.

It was time to call my mom. I knew this would probably be one of the most heartbreaking phone calls of my life. Like most mothers, my mom had dedicated her life to her family. She gave birth to me at age eighteen, and our family had been her world ever since.

My family had been through devastation and more trauma than most people could manage. When I was thirteen, I underwent tonsil surgery that went wrong. It resulted in a massive bleeding episode, and I almost bled to death. My siblings had their own medical issues. Rarely did a few months go by when one of us wasn't in the hospital for one thing or another.

"Why are my children always trying to die?" Mom would say. There were so many times when she thought she might lose one of us. And now I was about to tell her that I had cancer.

"Mom?" As she answered my video call, tears were already welling up in my eyes.

"Hun, what's wrong?"

"You know how I told you I was having my boob looked at?"

"Yeah?" The tears were now welling up in her eyes, too, as she scrunched her nose. Her heart already knew.

"It's cancer." I couldn't believe I got the words out.

Mom began to hyperventilate. Her eyes widened, and her breathing was fast and jagged. I could see the wheels turning in her brain as she wondered how this could be.

"Wait, wait," she said as she tried to make sense of the words that had just come from my mouth. "How do they know? Are they sure? How do they know?"

My dad and sister joined my mom in the dining room. It was past nine o'clock at night on the East Coast, and they had already turned in for the evening.

"I had a biopsy, and it was positive for cancer."

My mom and I were crying. Her eyes, unable to focus, darted around the room, desperate and panicked. My dad pulled out a chair and sat behind her, putting a hand on her shoulder. His brow furrowed. My dad wasn't a worrier. When I was a kid and had jumped from bed to bed in a hotel room and gashed my chin open, he insisted I didn't need stitches. He was of the mindset that everything would be fine. He always thought everything would turn out fine. But now, I could see that this was a different story.

"They're sure? Like, 100 percent? Are they sure? How are they sure?" My mom must have asked if they were sure and how they knew at least twenty times. She was looking for any hope that it wasn't true.

"Yes, they're sure," I told her.

Jonathan handed me my notebook where I had written down the conversation with the nurse. We were right to assume that we wouldn't remember anything on our own.

I read my notes and tried my best to explain the details to my mom, emphasizing the positive points, still trying to protect her from fear. "It has these hormone receptors, but she said that this type responds well to treatment."

Even in sharing one of the worst pieces of news someone could get, I was trying to protect my parents. They had both experienced tremendous amounts of loss in recent years. Several close family members had passed away suddenly and tragically. I didn't want them to think it was going to happen to me, too. I wanted to protect their hearts as much as I could.

Mom took notes in her own notebook as I read from mine. We talked about what the next steps were. I told her that the hospital was going to call the next day to get all my appointments set up.

"Will you need chemo?" she asked.

"I think so, yes," I replied. "But they said I'll find out more when I see the oncologist."

"I need to come take care of you. Tell Jonathan I'm moving in." Her plan to move to Utah was officially in motion.

CHAPTER 8
CALM BEFORE THE STORM

THE NEXT DAY, Jonathan stayed home from work. I cried all morning. My eyes were a leaky faucet that just couldn't be turned off. The tears kept coming and coming uncontrollably. Sometimes I sobbed, feeling wrung out, like every tear had taken my last bit of energy with it. Sometimes I cried silently as I tried to preoccupy myself with normal life tasks. I showered, fed the cats, and made breakfast. Tears dripped into the food, and I couldn't see clearly enough to use a knife.

"Let's go for a drive," Jonathan suggested.

"A drive? Where?" I asked.

"To your favorite tree."

The year before, when the world was locked down and everyone was social distancing thanks to the pandemic, Jonathan and I found a beautiful park in a nearby town. There were walking paths and trails through the forest. Situated on a small hill next to one of the paths was a gorgeous oak tree. Its branches hung down, engulfing its visitors in nature's hug. A bench sat under the branches, and I could stay there for hours if time allowed.

We got to the park, and I stepped out of the car. Although it was January, the weather was on the warmer side that afternoon. A light breeze hit my cheek and stopped me in my tracks. *Isn't it so amazing to be alive?*

I had never had a thought about what life means in any profound way before. But in that moment, an intense and sudden appreciation for life consumed me. Not that I didn't appreciate life before. I certainly did. But this was next-level. I cherished the cold on my face, the pockets of snow still on the ground from the last snowfall, the sounds of birds and bugs chirping, and the crunching leaves under my feet. Instead of overlooking every small thing, I felt like I was experiencing the world for the first time.

We made our way down the path to my favorite tree and sat on the bench under her branches. We stayed silent for a while, taking in the beauty of nature and this beautiful place in which we lived.

At a grouping of boulders in the center of the park, some children were playing a made-up game similar to The Floor Is Lava, jumping from rock to rock. People walked their dogs on the paved path. A squirrel scurried past us under the tree to gather an acorn left on the ground.

Had I never noticed these things before? Or had I just not paid this much attention? Why didn't anybody talk about these tiny pleasures in life? It felt like life had been superficial until this point. All the focus on unimportant details distracted from true meaning and joy.

"I've been thinking," I turned to Jonathan. "I think I need to be open about this and start telling people what's going on. It's going to be too hard to tell everybody one-on-one. I just can't do it."

"OK. What do you want to do then?"

"I think we should tell people closest to us first, like close friends and family. Then I'm going to post on social media. I don't want this to be a secret. I mean, people are going to find out anyway. It might as well be from me."

"That's true. You don't want people to hear it through the grapevine and wonder what the hell is going on."

"Right. It's not like I'm ashamed of it. I want to be open and honest about what we're going through. It might be nice to have extra support, too."

"Yeah, I agree."

I knew people who had gone through cancer treatment in the past and chose to keep it a secret. They wore wigs to hide their hair loss. They kept their medical appointments to themselves. While I understood the desire to look and appear as normal as possible to others, that wasn't my frame of mind. I didn't have family or friends nearby. It was just Jonathan and me. If I wanted support, and if I wanted my family to have the support they needed as well, I needed to tell people what was happening.

We continued to sit. Once the cat was out of the bag, everyone would know the truth. But for now, I could sit under my tree and pretend that life was perfect. At least for a few more hours.

CHAPTER 9
NOT FROM THIS

LATER THAT EVENING, I called a handful of close friends first. Then I drafted a post to share on social media. I couldn't mentally handle telling everyone individually. That would have been far too exhausting—like texting and calling every single person you know on Christmas morning to say Merry Christmas, except not as jolly and more like "Hey, just wanted to tell you I might die." It was just too much.

I paired my words with a photo Jonathan had taken of me in the park. I was wearing a black winter hat, complete with a pom-pom on top, and my black puffer coat. Even through my thick winter coat, it was recognizable that my left boob was bigger than the right. The problem was becoming more and more obvious.

Hey, friends. I want you to hear this from me, and not through the grapevine later on. I have breast cancer.

I debated how much to share, but I've decided to share openly. I'm not looking for pity. My hope in sharing is to receive all the prayers I can get. I also hope that sharing may help someone else.

I'm 35 years old and found it by doing a self-exam.

This really came out of the blue. I don't smoke or drink alcohol. I eat a healthy, whole foods diet. I practice mindfulness.

I'm a health hippie. I don't know of anyone in my biological family who has had breast cancer. I was considered "low risk."

Around the holidays, I noticed a change in my left side. I thought little of it because I gained some weight during 2020, and boobs grow with weight gain, right? After the new year, it started feeling sore. I did a self-exam and found a lump.

Last Friday, I had a mammogram and ultrasound. They found a mass the size of a dime, and a nearby lymph node was larger than it should be. I had multiple biopsies that same day.

Four days later, I was diagnosed with invasive ductal carcinoma in my breast and lymph node. It hasn't been assigned a stage yet because I need more testing first. I've been told that this type of cancer responds well to treatment.

I will meet with my oncology team this week and undergo lots of additional testing. They'll assign it a stage, and we'll go from there with surgery and treatment options.

I won't lie and pretend like I'm just A-OK with it all. I'm not. I've done a lot of crying. Every day is an emotional roller coaster right now. Sometimes I have hope, sometimes massive dread and fear. Even though I'm scared as hell, I am hopeful that I'll heal from this cancer.

I intend to follow the guidance of my medical team, both with treatment options and holistic support. I am putting my whole heart and soul into healing. I have to.

I'll be treated at the Huntsman Cancer Institute in Salt Lake City. Everyone there has been great so far.

I have a good support system. We're supported by our military family here. And although far away, we have the love and support of our family and friends.

If you know Jonathan, please check on him through this process. He's the strongest, most capable person I know, but I worry about him stoically taking on too much. (He knows I worry about this.)

If you're the spiritual type, I accept all prayers, healing vibes, good juju, positivity, whatever your thing is. I believe in the power of positive intention, especially in big numbers. This is something I greatly need.

Please. Please. No matter your health habits, age, gender, race, whatever, PLEASE FEEL YOUR BOOBIES! Get to know your body so you'll know if something changes. Look at yourself in the mirror. If you've been avoiding a mammogram, schedule it ASAP. Please.

I'm not really sure how to end this. This feels weird. But if you've read this whole thing, thank you.

I'll update as I feel able.

I love you.

Feel your boobies.

I published the post and turned off my phone. Telling the world somehow made it feel real, and I wasn't emotionally ready for the response. I was scared of what people might say. I didn't want anyone to treat me differently. I didn't want pity. I didn't want to be treated like a corpse in waiting. I didn't want any of that. I wanted everyone to treat me like the same Emily. Because I was the same. Just with cancer. So I left my phone off for the night.

In bed that night, I was a sobbing mess. It seems like difficult things become even more difficult after the sun goes down. Fear crept in. I felt out of control not knowing how bad my situation truly was and how it would be treated. The unknown was the scariest part.

Jonathan wrapped his arms around me as I spiraled mentally and emotionally, sobbing and wailing so loudly that I'm sure the neighbors heard.

"I can't do this," I said through hyperventilating breaths. "I can't do this. I don't know how I'm going to handle this. I don't think my body can do it. I think I'm going to die. I know I'm going to die. I should just die now and get it over with so I don't have to suffer."

"Fish, take a breath." Jonathan had affectionately called me Fish since our dating days because my pursed, kissing lips looked like a fish's mouth. How romantic.

"I can't. I can't. I don't want to. I just want to die and get it over with." I was hyperventilating and could barely breathe. Fear consumed my brain.

"Please, just give it until morning. Do it for me. If you can't do it for yourself, please do it for me. Just until morning."

I reluctantly agreed. I could at least get through until morning, even if I was convinced that one night wouldn't change anything.

I'm not sure how I fell asleep that night, but somehow I did.

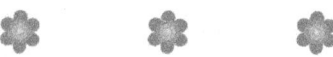

My Uncle Keith passed away in early 2014 in a snowmobile accident. It was sudden, tragic, and devastating to our family. He was the best uncle in the world—always there for me and always supportive. After he passed away, I received signs from his spirit, but nothing that couldn't be passed off as a coincidence. A song on the radio that he liked. Hearing someone in public with a similar voice. It happened every so often, and I was reminded of him.

While I was dreaming that night, I thought I was awake. That's how clear it was. I was walking down a bright corridor when Uncle Keith approached me and gave me a big bear hug. He didn't feel alive. I knew he was dead. But we were there together in a very real place. His hug felt as real as a hug could feel.

If he's dead, I thought, *he must have gone to the spirit world. And that means he knows things. This is my chance to ask him questions.*

Not wanting to waste time, I asked him bluntly, "Is this how I die? From this cancer?"

"Not from this," he said. "Not from this."

I felt the most relieving sigh exit my body as I opened my eyes. I was in my bedroom in Utah, with morning sunlight peeking through the blinds. The words repeated in my head.

Not from this.

CHAPTER 10

BLANKETS

A MENTOR ONCE told me that the best way to offer help is to be specific.

Can I make dinner for your family on Thursday?

Can I bring napkins to the party?

Would you like me to take care of your cat while you're in the hospital?

"When people are going through a difficult time," she said, "they don't know what they need. Especially if they've never gone through that thing before."

It wasn't until this moment that I fully understood what she meant. I didn't know what I wanted to eat for dinner, let alone what I needed to survive cancer.

After I posted my announcement on social media, the floodgates opened. Everyone wanted to know what they could do to help. And I had no idea. I didn't know what I needed. I'd never done this before.

The only thing I could think about was Jonathan and the help he would need. For our entire marriage, I had done most of the household tasks—cooking, cleaning, paying bills, taking care of the pets, coordinating home and car maintenance, all the things. We were equal partners, but that's the life of a military spouse, especially during deployments and long duty days.

I was used to being alone and doing everything myself. All those responsibilities would now fall on his shoulders.

At the same time, Jonathan was a capable person. There was nothing he couldn't figure out. I knew he'd figure out how to balance work and our household. But I questioned the toll it would take on his emotional and mental well-being. I knew he would wear himself to the ground to take care of me. *It's my responsibility as a husband*, he would say. *It's my job.*

I asked friends and family to check in on Jonathan and make sure he was handling everything OK. I knew he'd lie and say that everything was fine, that he didn't need help. And he'd probably believe it to be true. But I wanted him to be reminded that there were people who cared and were waiting in the wings to catch him.

When it came to what I would need help with, I was at a loss. I wasn't sure how anyone could help me. The only thing I wanted was to feel less alone. Cancer is a lonely place. Ultimately, I was the only one who would experience the hell of treatment. I was the one who would be kept in isolation due to a weakened immune system. But I didn't want to feel alone.

I asked for friends and family to be there if I needed someone to talk to, to complain to about treatment when I was feeling like a steaming pile of poo, or to just shoot the breeze with when I needed a distraction. I needed people to help me feel normal through the most abnormal time of my life.

When I say people came through, they really came through.

If I had a dollar for every prayer, every message of well-wishes, every ounce of love I felt, I could buy a nice vacation. Maybe even a first-class plane ticket to go with it.

My favorite thing about the military community is knowing people from all over the world. Prayers and positive energy flowed from every corner of the earth. I felt overwhelmed and unable to process what was happening. But I was grateful for every bit.

"Our prayer group in Thailand is praying for you."

"I lit a candle for you at Notre Dame."

"I'd like to send you energy for a strengthened immune system."

"I know we haven't talked in a long time, but I'm thinking of you."

If you know much about *The Five Love Languages* by Gary Chapman, you know about how people give and receive love. My primary love language is "words of affirmation," and words of encouragement were especially meaningful. I received many nonphysical gifts, a result of the digital age we live in. Memes and jokes lifted my spirits. They say laughter is the best medicine after all.

Friends and family sent physical gifts, too. They anticipated what I needed without me having to use my limited energy to ask for it. Packages flooded my front porch. There were handwritten notes, drawings from children (my favorite was one from my friend's daughter, a sketch of me kicking a butt—cancer's butt), meal delivery gift cards, snacks, cozy socks, fun nail art supplies, notebooks, pillows, and so much more. But nothing compared to the gift everyone thought I needed most: blankets.

I received eleven blankets in total. Fuzzy blankets, custom blankets with pictures of my cats on them, weighted blankets, blankets printed with inspirational words, and handmade crocheted blankets. In college, I had taught my best friend how to crochet. When I was diagnosed, she crocheted me a blanket. It was a full-circle moment that filled my heart with pride and joy.

Receiving so many gifts was a reminder of how much I was loved. And how cold everyone thought I was. But I mostly felt incredibly loved.

CHAPTER 11
I DID EVERYTHING RIGHT

I SAW THE LAST of my Reiki clients a week after my diagnosis. I knew it would be too difficult to do Reiki sessions while undergoing treatment. I wouldn't be able to stand for an hour at a time, and I would need to devote every bit of the energy I had going toward healing my own body.

"I need to temporarily close my Reiki studio," I told my clients. "I have cancer, and I need this time to heal." I made sure to use the word *temporarily*. I didn't want them to think I was abandoning them or that I didn't intend to return. And subconsciously, I think I was telling myself that I'd make it through this. Reiki was my calling. It brought me joy. It was one of my life purposes. I had every intention of returning. If I lived, so would my practice. That was my intention.

Saying these words, telling my clients I had cancer, felt embarrassing. Here I was, a Reiki Master, someone who helped other people with their ailments—physical, emotional, and spiritual—and I got cancer. I was supposed to be someone people looked up to in terms of health and balance. I know now that was my ego speaking, but it felt embarrassing at the time, like I didn't have my shit together.

In the energy healing community, cancer is thought to be a side effect of some deeper, unaddressed imbalance. Some people think that if you're energetically balanced, there's no way you can get cancer. "It's the cancer-free way," I've been told.

I'm here to formally announce that it's bullshit and untrue for several reasons. I don't think anyone is truly 100 percent "balanced." Everyone has a thing, something in their life that is stressful or traumatic. Everyone is human. We're all just people. Telling someone they won't get cancer if they just do everything "right" is downright toxic. People think they can control life, but life, by its very nature, is uncontrollable in so many ways.

I used to believe that if you took care of your body and spirit, disease wouldn't be able to thrive, that the body would be incompatible with disease. That's what I was taught. I now believe that disease is random. Cancer is simply a group of wonky cells that quickly replicate.

I had done everything right. I meditated daily. I received Reiki and bodywork from other professionals. I was physically active and fit. I ate a mostly organic diet of real whole foods. I hadn't consumed processed sugar in ten years. You read that right. Ten years. How, you might ask? I was incredibly self-disciplined, health-focused, and under the impression that being sugar-free was how one created true health.

While I was over here being a health nut, my genetics were doing everything right, too. A blood test showed that I had no known genetic markers for any type of cancer. I had no family history of breast cancer. Good genes were on my side.

I was under the impression that I was completely healthy. And yet, I wasn't. I still got cancer. An unhealthy lifestyle and genetic mutations can lead to disease, but living a healthy lifestyle and having good genes won't prevent it. Anything can happen to anyone.

After I saw my last client before the whirlwind of treatment would begin, Jonathan approached me with an idea for the Reiki studio. "What do you think about dismantling it to make more room for your mom?" One of the extra rooms in our home had become my Reiki studio when I opened my practice. I loved seeing clients in my home studio. It was cozy, the privacy made my clients feel comfortable and safe, and I didn't have to pay rent.

"As much as it hurts my heart," I said, "I think you're right."

My mom would be moving in in a few weeks, and we decided to move some of the bedrooms around to make the most use of our space. I wanted her to have her own private area of the house, a bedroom with a dedicated bathroom on the second floor.

One day when Jonathan had the day off from work, we took apart the Reiki room and moved everything to the unfinished basement. I folded up the treatment table, dismantled the ambient lighting, boxed up my books, and took art off the walls. Jonathan hoisted the blush pink client couch over his back and carried it down two flights of stairs by himself. He didn't want me doing any physical labor. I packed the boxes, and he carried them.

It was heartbreaking to watch my career—the long-awaited career that had barely gotten started—go into storage. The pink couch was the heart of the studio. It was the bright smile and warm hug that enveloped my clients as we talked about their hopes, desires, and lives.

"It's just temporary," Jonathan said as a tear rolled down my face. "You'll be back to doing Reiki when you're well, and it'll be even better than before."

I hoped that was true. Until then, the pink couch, along with my source of joy, my offering to the world, would hibernate on a cold concrete floor covered in an old bed sheet, gathering dust.

CHAPTER 12
A RARITY

TIME CAN BE a cruel thing. The week between the diagnosis call and when I saw a doctor was nothing short of mental torture. Knowing something bad was happening but not having a plan yet was driving me a little bonkers.

My first stop on the cancer treatment train was the breast surgeon. Dr. R., my assigned surgeon, was a petite woman with curly graying hair. Although small in stature, she walked into the room with a commanding presence. Following introductions, she said something that caught me off guard.

"Do you know why you're here?" she asked in a quiet, soft voice while sitting on a swivel stool next to me.

I wondered if she meant this in a spiritual sense. *Well*, I thought, *I have no idea anymore. I actually don't know much of anything, to be honest.* Or did she mean this in a literal sense, as in, do I know why I'm sitting in an exam room at a cancer hospital?

"Um, because I have cancer?" I hoped the obvious answer was the correct one.

"So you know that it's cancer. Some people make it to this point and still don't realize they have cancer."

"Yes, I know I have cancer, but I'm going to be OK." I knew I'd be OK because of my dream, but I wasn't about to tell the doctor that part. *Yeah, I know I won't die because my dead uncle said so.* I'd surely sound unhinged.

Dr. R looked at me with pity in her eyes. "It's good to have a positive attitude," she said with the gentlest bedside manner and a pat on my leg. "A positive mindset is important for healing." I sensed that she wasn't as sure as I was. "Let's go through everything we know so far so we can make a plan moving forward with treatment."

She sat close to me, whipped out a piece of paper with breast diagrams on it, and reviewed every detail that was found in my biopsy. My brain had been fried in a pan of medical terminology for the last week, and I appreciated her use of layperson's terms.

"Your tumor is located about here." She circled an area on a side portrait of a hand-drawn breast. "It's about the size of a dime right now." She drew sketches and doodles of milk ducts, breast tissue, and lymph nodes, illustrating what she thought was happening inside me.

Jonathan sat in a chair in the corner of the room, feverishly taking notes in the trusty notebook. He wrote down every detail because we knew it would be impossible to remember them later, just as it was with the initial call.

"Now let's talk about a plan for treating this. Do you guys have children?"

"Not yet," I replied.

"Do you ever plan to have biological children?"

Jonathan and I looked at each other, not sure what to say. We had always had the mindset that if we got pregnant by chance, we'd be OK with it, but we weren't actively trying to get pregnant.

"I ask because if you are, we need to send you to fertility before you begin treatment. Is this something you want to do?" she continued.

"What would that mean for treatment?" I asked.

"Well, it would delay it a little bit."

Jonathan and I looked at each other again. We had been together since we were teenagers and could just about read each other's minds by now. Many conversations happened in silence.

Me: It would delay treatment.
Jonathan: Do you want to do it?
Me: I don't think so. Are you OK with that?
Jonathan: I'm OK with it.

Jonathan gave a slight shake of his head.

"No, we're not going to do fertility." That was it. In three seconds, one of the biggest decisions of our lives was made. We were never going to have biological children.

Dr. R looked relieved. "OK, that's probably a good idea so you can start treatment as soon as possible. I just want to make sure that you're sure."

I was sure. Given the option of having children but delaying treatment and the cancer possibly spreading or staying barren and alive, I'd choose the latter every single time.

"I'm going to let you change." Dr. R. stood up to leave the room. "And I'll be back to take a look at what we can see."

Meredith, her nurse, handed me a gown. I changed into it and climbed onto the exam table.

When she returned, Dr. R looked intently at each of my breasts. She examined them and pressed on them the way doctors do when they're giving a breast exam. Thank God she didn't try to pop my nipple. I didn't need that again.

"Have you ever heard of inflammatory breast cancer?" she asked.

Oh no, I thought. I *had* heard of IBC a few years earlier while consulting the internet on something unrelated during a trip down the Dr. Google rabbit hole. Everything I had read about it was terrifying.

"Actually, yes," I said, remembering the orange-peel appearance of the breasts I had seen online. "Why? Does my boob look like that?"

"It could be. It could also be advanced lymphatic involvement, but we'll need an MRI to tell for sure. Do you mind if I bring some nurses in to look at your breast? This could be a good learning experience for them." The University of Utah, which includes Huntsman Cancer Institute, is a teaching hospital. Medical students are often silent shadows in the corners of clinic exam rooms.

If my wonky boob could be a learning experience, then I was OK with that. A line of nurses soon entered the room, each bending over to look closer at my boobs. I stayed silent while feeling like a rare, endangered animal being oohed and aahed over at the zoo.

"Wow," one said in breathy amazement. "Yeah, I see that."

See what? What did she see?

As Dr. R. pointed out my swollen breast to the nurses, indicating its color and shape, I had a sinking feeling that IBC was a very real possibility and quickly got over feeling offended by everyone being in awe of my bosom. The feeling soon turned to terror welling up in my chest. Then worry. If this was so rare that they'd never seen something like this before, I wondered if the doctors here knew how to treat it. It was a real concern.

"Have you ever treated IBC before?" I bluntly asked Dr. R as the final nurse left the room.

"Yes. Not incredibly often, but we have, yes. If it is IBC, though, surgery won't be your first stop. IBC patients go to medical oncology first for chemo, then surgery. I'm going to order you a pretreatment chest MRI, and that will tell us for sure what's going on and if it's inflammatory breast cancer."

Meredith found an open slot and scheduled me for a chest MRI the next day.

CHAPTER 13
SCANXIETY

THE NEXT MORNING, I put on a pair of big gold hoop earrings, my new go-to look for feeling semi-normal.

"Are you sure you want to wear those?" Jonathan asked. "You're just going to have to take everything off anyway, especially metal."

"You're right." I took off the earrings and left them at home.

Jonathan and I drove to the hospital bright and early. The air was clear, a rare sight for Utah in the winter. The inversion, a weather phenomenon that traps a layer of smog on the valley floor, typically plagues the Salt Lake area this time of year. Even so, I could barely appreciate the crisp, cool air. My nerves were shot from the emotions I was feeling since being diagnosed. I was in a constant state of anxiety.

"Emily?" someone called as they opened the door to the waiting area. This was becoming familiar. I took off my wedding rings and handed them to Jonathan to put on his pinkie finger.

"You'll do great," he said firmly, kissing me before I went back for my scan.

I was learning that it was best to wear shirts that slipped off easily when changing into a hospital gown. Bras were optional, and with how painful my boob had become in the weeks prior, I often didn't wear one.

"Do you have any jewelry on?" the radiologist asked, scanning my earlobes, neck, and fingers before taking me into the MRI room.

"No, I took everything off," I said as we made small talk while walking toward the machine.

"You can just lie face down right here."

I noticed there were two holes in the table. "Um, excuse me? Do my boobs go in those holes?" I had never put my boobs in holes before and didn't want to get it wrong. The embarrassment of my boobs ending up someplace they shouldn't be would plague me for eternity. I'd think about it every day for the rest of my life.

"Yes, and your face goes on that rest just like a massage table."

As I lay there, boobs hanging low and arms reaching above my head, she put a set of headphones over my ears. Being inside the MRI machine feels like being in a coffin, and claustrophobia can kick in fast, so they offer music to keep people from freaking out. She placed an emergency button in my hand just in case I panicked in the coffin tube and needed to abort mission.

"I see you requested . . . Hanson?"

"Yes. They're my favorite."

I began an "MMMBop" dance party in my head and didn't hit the emergency button once.

CHAPTER 14

SATURDAY MORNING

AT EIGHT O'CLOCK in the morning, I got a call from an unknown number. I almost didn't answer it, especially so early on a Saturday morning. Because of my East Coast area code, spam calls and time zones weren't my friend. But I answered anyway.

"Emily, this is Dr. R," the voice on the other end said. "I'm sorry to bother you so early on a Saturday. Are you and your husband available to talk?"

Jonathan rushed into the kitchen, grabbing his notebook en route. I sat at the kitchen island and pressed the speaker phone button.

"OK, we're ready."

"We got the MRI results back, and it looks like there is cancer diffused throughout the breast tissue."

"What does that mean?" I asked.

"Well, it could be one of two things. It could be inflammatory breast cancer, like we talked about, or it could be advanced lymphatic involvement. Sometimes when the lymph node is positive for cancer, it blocks the lymphatic flow through the breast tissue and can clog those pathways. I think we talked about that on Thursday."

I still didn't understand the difference. "What does this mean for me? And at what point can we tell if it's IBC or not?"

I was still trying to have hope that it wasn't IBC. IBC was scary. The statistics were scary. I didn't want that. I wanted the lymph clogging thing.

"I'm making the clinical diagnosis now," Dr. R said. "It's safe to say you have inflammatory breast cancer."

My heart dropped into my toes. Time stopped. Earth's spin halted. I had inflammatory breast cancer.

CHAPTER 15
MAKING A PLAN

I HUNG UP the phone and flung my arms around Jonathan. "It's the bad one." I wrapped myself around him and buried my face in his chest. He held me close, not saying anything.

I hadn't wanted to admit it, but in my heart, I already knew it was IBC. With how inflamed and sore my boob had become, I didn't know how it couldn't be. My left breast was so painful that I could no longer sleep on that side. And forget about sleeping on my stomach. Hearing the news from Dr. R. was simply validation that my intuition was correct, even if my brain didn't want to believe it.

Everything I knew about IBC was bad—the aggressiveness of the cancer and how quickly it could spread throughout the body. I had read that it could be a matter of weeks before it became metastatic. I was now thankful that we'd forgone fertility treatments. That decision would save my life.

"Am I going to be OK?" I asked Jonathan as I looked up into his eyes, tears streaming down my face.

"You're gonna be OK," he said, lying through his teeth. I didn't believe him. I wanted the comfort of hearing those words, but I didn't believe them. Plus, he had his "deer in headlights" look. When Jonathan is overwhelmed, his eyes widen and he stares forward, unable to focus. I could see that he was scared.

I was scared, too. I needed to lean on the message from Uncle Keith now more than ever. He said I wouldn't die from this. To get through this fear, I had to believe him.

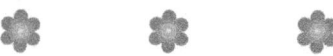

On Tuesday morning, a week later, we arrived at the same clinic where we had met Dr. R. We were led into the same room where I had felt like a zoo exhibit. Déjà vu.

The medical oncologist, a petite woman with round glasses and curly salt-and-pepper hair, walked in. I wondered if all oncology doctors had a similar look.

"Emily? I'm Dr. B." Her voice was warm and commanded the room. At the same time, it soothed our nerves. She walked over to me and took my hands in hers. I didn't know this woman, but her energy was a nurturing hug. I had trouble trusting medical providers since I'd nearly bled to death from tonsil surgery as a child. But when Dr. B held my hands as she looked into my eyes, smiled, and gave a reassuring nod, I felt trust.

Dr. B shook Jonathan's hand and introduced us to her nurse, Rachel. She asked a lot of questions, and we talked about everything that had led to this point. Rachel stood at the computer, typing away, as Dr. B occasionally huddled in to give her notes. They pointed at the screen, collaborating like a well-oiled machine. They were in sync with each other's thoughts.

"I took a look at your MRI results from last week, and I agree with Dr. R that this is inflammatory breast cancer," she said, rolling her stool closer to me. "I think it's a good idea to begin chemotherapy as soon as possible. With IBC, the protocol is to receive chemo first, then surgery, then radiation. There may be more treatment after that, but we'll take one step at a time." Dr. B took out a notepad and started writing down the steps to a proposed treatment plan.

"First will be the chemo." Dr. B spoke in an academic tone, but her body language showed motherly care. Her voice sounded like that of a favorite professor. "And we have to get you scheduled to have a port put in as soon as possible." Having a port—a device placed just under the skin on the non-cancer side of the chest—put in would be a minor surgery.

"A connected tube will go up into your neck, into your jugular vein," she continued. "When they give you chemo or other medication, they can just give it right through that port instead of having to poke you with IVs every time." That sounded much easier than having my elbow pit stabbed in search of a vein with every trip to the clinic. I was Team Port already. "And I think that TCHP will be the best chemo option for you."

"I'm looking at that now," Rachel chimed in. "And I agree."

"It's a good option for cancer that's triple positive. It's a combination of four medications: Taxotere, Carboplatin, Herceptin, and Perjeta. The Herceptin and Perjeta will target the HER2 receptor, giving us our best chance at a cure. The Taxotere and Carboplatin are systemic drugs that target any cancer cells throughout the body."

"I'm sorry, hold on," I interrupted. "Did you say cure? Do you think this is curable?"

"I'm going to send you for a PET scan to make sure, but nothing in your MRI indicated that this has spread beyond your lymph nodes. The rest of the chest area looks clear, but we'll scan the whole body to check everything else."

"So if it hasn't spread further," I pressed, "it's curable? Do people become cured from inflammatory breast cancer?"

"It's totally curable. As long as it's stage III. But we're taking it one step at a time. We'll be able to stage you properly after the PET scan when we know everything going on."

Totally curable. I'd hang on to that phrase for a long time, even though I knew that there was no real cure for cancer. What she meant was that there was a chance that my body could one day be free of cancer. There's a difference.

She was realistic and didn't mince words. She didn't give me false hope. But at that moment, the tiniest sliver of hope was all I needed. Tears flowed uncontrollably as Jonathan dug through my purse in search of a tissue. This was the first time I'd heard this level of optimism from anyone besides Uncle Keith's spirit.

"Oh my God," I sobbed. "I'm so happy. I promise I'm going to do my best. I didn't know if it could ever be cured because I've been googling IBC and—"

"Whoa, whoa." She put my rambling to a halt with the look of a disappointed mother. "You've been googling? Why do you want to put yourself in jail?"

"Put myself in jail? What do you mean?"

"The internet is scary. Stay off it. And the information on there is old anyway. The medications we use now are different, and protocols have changed. We're seeing much better results now. It's best to stay off Google. Look at me." She bent over to look into my eyes. "Promise you'll stay off the internet?"

"I promise," I sniffled. She gave a curt nod and went back to the notepad detailing my treatment timeline.

"After the six rounds of chemo, you'll get a short break to get your blood counts closer to normal, then you'll have surgery with Dr. R. She's really great. Surgery will be either a single or a double mastectomy. Then you'll have radiation. But that's in a long time, so don't worry about that just yet."

"Is radiation the end of treatment then?" I asked.

"Well, kind of, but not really. If the pathology from your surgery shows that all the cancer is gone, you'll stay on just Herceptin for a few more months. But if pathology shows that chemo didn't kill all the cancer, you'll have Kadcyla, which is Herceptin combined with another chemotherapy drug."

She drew a diagram like a flowchart you'd see in a textbook. If this happens, then here's an arrow to go over here. And if that happens, follow this arrow over there. Choose your own adventure. Or rather, the pathology will choose your adventure for you. I loved those types of books as a kid. Now I was living the real-life version—the cancer edition.

"More chemo?" I asked. I looked to Jonathan for support, but his face was full of overwhelm, unsure how to make sense of the amount of information flying at us. We both looked to Dr. B in unison.

"Yes, but it's targeted chemo. So it won't be as intense as TCHP. But we don't even know if you'll need that, so we'll take it as it comes." It seemed she was a big fan of taking things as they come. I, on the other hand, needed to know every possible path and possibility before beginning the journey.

"And that's all after radiation?"

"It'll be at the same time. Radiation and targeted therapy will occur simultaneously."

Looking at everything yet to come was overwhelming. According to the timeline, treatment would take more than a year. I prepared for it to consume my life. I prepared to make the hospital my second home for the next year. As difficult as treatment would be, I was thankful to have a plan, a timeline to wrap my head around. I found comfort in knowing what was about to happen and what would happen next. I found myself entering "mission mode." I pushed my fear and complicated feelings to the side momentarily and prepared for the most important mission of my life: to become "totally cured."

CHAPTER 16
SKINNY NECK

MY HOUR WITH DR. B ended, and Rachel stayed behind to go over my schedule. The next week would be the busiest yet. There'd be no more sitting around and waiting anymore. There was action, and I was stoked about getting the ball rolling.

"So you'll get your port next week," she said.

"Is that scary, getting that thing put under my skin?" I asked. "Will I be awake for it?"

A friend who had gone through breast cancer several years earlier warned me about having a port placed. "Make sure they knock you out. I was awake, and it was the most traumatic experience of my life." This came from a woman who had given birth multiple times.

"I think you'll have the option," Rachel explained. "But you won't remember it either way. They'll give you sleepy drugs, and you'll just be like . . ." She rolled her eyes back in her head, stuck out her tongue slightly, and bobbed her head up and down as if pretending to be drunk.

At the University of Utah's outpatient surgery center a few days later, I met the surgeon and anesthesiologist who'd be placing my port.

"Can I be asleep for the procedure?" I asked the anesthesiologist.

"If you want, sure. Recovery time will be a little longer, but we can definitely put you under general anesthesia if that's what you'd like."

"Yes, that's what I'd like," I said, no longer timid to express my medical preferences. The anesthesiologist left, and the surgeon stayed behind to explain what was going to happen.

"We're just going to make two little incisions, one on your chest and one on your neck so we can guide the tube up into your jugular. You have a skinny neck, so it'll be really easy."

I was slightly overweight and was sure nobody had ever called my neck skinny before, except for that one bully in elementary school who called me Pencil Neck on the school bus. She tried to hurt my feelings, but little did she know that my neck would make my life "really easy" one day. Take that.

"When we're done," the surgeon continued, "you'll come back here to your hubby while you wake up. Then you'll go home, and I'll see you again when you get it taken out."

Before long, a nurse came to roll me to the operating room. "Did they give you Valium?" he asked.

"No," I said as he wheeled me down the hallway. "I haven't had anything yet."

"You're the calmest person I've ever taken back to surgery." I was feeling pretty calm. I just wanted it to be over. And I was praying I wouldn't remember anything.

When I opened my eyes, I was back in the patient room where Jonathan was waiting.

"Hi, love," he said. "You're all done. You did great."

"Is it in?" I asked.

"Yup. Everything went great."

A week later, I'd find out that everything, in fact, was not great.

CHAPTER 17
FIRST CHEMO

JONATHAN PARKED the car in one of the spots at the Huntsman infusion center reserved for patients. It was eight o'clock in the morning, and I was about to receive my first chemotherapy treatment, my first round of TCHP. Jonathan's arms were full, carrying his backpack, his work bag, my purse, and my giant tote bag full of activities to keep my mind busy for the day. I held a fluffy pink blanket gifted to me by my friend Angela. It was the first of the famous eleven blankets. We were a sight to see.

"Welcome." The woman behind the check-in desk had a cheerful voice.

"Don't mind us," I joked. "We're moving in for the day."

"That's perfectly fine. Have a seat, and they'll call you back shortly."

We sat in the waiting area, our stuff taking up two seats of its own. Putting it all down felt like a mistake when we had to pick it all back up a minute later.

"Emily?" a pretty woman with long, thick dark hair called to me from the doorway leading to the infusion area. "I'm Jackie. I'll be taking care of you today."

She led us to the large, sterile, and intimidating infusion room full of medical equipment and nursing staff. Big vinyl chairs were separated into pods by hospital curtains. They looked kind of like those faux leather massage chairs you might see in the middle of the mall. Why anyone would want to have a massage in the middle of the mall with everyone watching was beyond me, but to each their own. IV poles with digital screens stood next to each chair. Each pod had one uncomfortable-looking plastic seat, presumably for the accompanying loved one.

"You guys are lucky," Jackie said. "They just started allowing one visitor last week." I did feel lucky, and my heart ached for every person who had to do this alone because of the pandemic protocols. I couldn't imagine going through all of this without Jonathan by my side.

"This is your first chemo, right?" Jackie asked.

"Yep. First one."

She led us to a nearby curtained-off pod. Jonathan set the mountain of stuff on the floor with a thud.

"It's a reclining massage chair," Jackie explained when I sat down in the big gray throne. "The controls are on the arm right there."

As I was playing around with the buttons, evaluating my options for how high I wanted to recline my legs, Jackie prepared me for what to expect.

"Do you have a port?" she asked.

"Yes." I unbuttoned the shoulder snaps on my shirt, which had been recommended by a woman in a social media group: "This is actually a maternity shirt meant for breastfeeding, but it's perfect for us chemo girls," she wrote. I bought one immediately. The top was held together by three snaps on each shoulder, and when unbuttoned, just enough of my chest was revealed to expose my port, allowing me to keep my shirt on for the infusion. It was late February and frigid outside. I didn't want to undress for this.

"That shirt is perfect," Jackie said. She poked and felt the bump under my skin. She paid close attention to the new incision. "Has your port been accessed before, or is this the first time?"

"This is the first time," I replied.

"It's super easy." Jackie opened a sterile package and put on a yellow paper gown. She laid out all the supplies in the pack—gauze, alcohol pads, an adhesive square, and the needle that would be inserted into my port. She talked me through it as she went through each step. It was as easy as she promised. Much easier than being poked in my elbow pit by an IV, hoping the needle had made it into a vein. With the adhesive square holding everything in place, there was now a clear tube dangling from my chest. It felt weird and made me officially feel like a sick cancer patient. I didn't like that feeling. If shit wasn't getting real before, it certainly was now.

"We'll get some blood drawn for labs first to make sure you're healthy enough to receive chemo today," Jackie said. "Then we'll get started. First will be your pre-meds—steroids and something to help with nausea. Those will help you tolerate the chemo better. Then we'll start the chemo. Because it's your first time, we'll need to wait in between each of the medications to make sure you don't have an allergic reaction. That's why today will take about nine hours."

Nine. Hours.

She took blood from my port, and I turned my head to look away. The sight of other people's blood didn't bother me, but when it came to my own, forget about it. I got woozy every time. I couldn't look.

When she was done, I opened my tote bag, took out my headphones, and opened up YouTube on my phone. I had recently been obsessed with videos of people walking around Disney parks, revealing park secrets and overlooked details that most people didn't notice. I loved Disney. My family took a vacation to Florida every other year while I was growing up, and the parks and movies were a huge part of my life. It was my favorite place, and the thought of possibly never going again was distressing. Jonathan and I went to Walt Disney World for our honeymoon and had returned many times. Watching these YouTube videos made me feel like I was there again and gave me hope that one day, I'd go back. One day, I would do "normal people" things again.

"Good news." Jackie opened the pod curtain and came in. "Your labs are perfect. We can get started."

After receiving the pre-meds consisting of steroids and anti-nausea medication and waiting for an allergic reaction that didn't come, it was time. Jackie called in another nurse to assist her as she put on what can only be described as a hazmat suit. This shit was so poisonous, the nurses wore hazmat suits. And this poison was about to go into my body, into my veins, into my cells.

Jackie read off the information printed on the IV bag full of chemotherapy, verifying with the other nurse who was reading from the computer screen that she had rolled into the room with her.

"Can you verify your name and date of birth?" Jackie asked. There were multiple checks to make sure they didn't give the wrong medication to the wrong patient. That would certainly be a nightmare. And a lawsuit.

I recited my legal government name followed by my date of birth.

"That's a long last name," she said. "How do you pronounce it again?"

My legal last name was a hot topic among medical staff and anyone else who had to read my ID card. I had chosen to hyphenate when we got married because I didn't want to make things more complicated than they needed to be by adopting an entirely new last name. However, in my attempt to prevent complications, I had somehow given myself one of the most complicated identities known to womankind, or so you'd think by the reactions I received.

Jackie hooked the first bag of chemotherapy to the machine and my port and hit the buttons to start the process. The IV pump whirred and dripped the medication into the tube.

"You know," Jackie said. "I had this same chemotherapy."

"*You* had chemotherapy?" I asked, looking at her thick, gorgeous hair. It was hard to believe that hair that beautiful came from her head after being so sick and bald.

"Yep. I had triple-positive breast cancer, too. Not inflammatory, but I also had TCHP. If you're interested, I can give you some recipes for the scalp oil and scalp shampoo I used." (*See Helpful Recipes section at the end.*)

"That would be amazing." I was still in awe that this woman, who had also been through hell, was here taking care of me as I began this journey. "Were you an infusion nurse before you had cancer?"

"No," she said. "I became a nurse afterward to help other

people going through it."

I will never be convinced that this woman was not an angel sent directly from heaven.

When I received the second bag of chemo, this one full of Carboplatin, it was time for lunch. There was a café in the clinic lobby. Jonathan left the infusion area to take a picture of the menu board and returned so I could choose what I wanted to eat.

"I think I'll have the chicken quesadilla," I said. "That sounds good." I loved Mexican food, especially quesadillas filled with grilled chicken and ooey-gooey cheese. My favorite.

Jonathan returned with lunch and laid out the container of food, cutlery, and napkin on my lap. I opened the to-go shell and took a bite of the quesadilla.

What. The. Hell. It was the grossest thing I had tasted in my life.

"Jonny, does this smell bad?" I handed him a piece of quesadilla.

He sniffed it and took a bite. "Seems OK to me," he said, handing it back to me.

"I'm so sorry, but I can't eat this. I thought it was going to be good, but it's not." I couldn't put my finger on *how* it tasted bad, but it just did. Jonathan ate the rest, and I opted for a couple of bags of the free pretzels from the nurse's station.

Seven hundred Disney videos and nine hours later, the IV pump beeped its final beep of the day, indicating that the last bag of chemo was empty. It was already five o'clock, and I was the last patient remaining in the building.

"You did it!" Jackie flung the curtain open. "One down, five to go. How are you feeling?"

"Good," I said. "Just tired, and my butt is sore from sitting." I couldn't wait to get unplugged from the IV pole and go home.

That was the last time I'd say I felt good for a very, very long time.

"Just one more thing before you leave. I need to put your Neulasta device on."

After every round of chemotherapy, I had a device stuck to the back of my arm. The medication inside, Neulasta, self-injected twenty-seven hours after being applied. Neulasta stimulates the immune system, encouraging the body to create more of a type of white blood cell called neutrophils. It does this by increasing the production of bone marrow, which can cause severe bone pain in the process.

After Jackie disconnected my port and the device was attached to my arm, Jonathan gathered all our bags, my blanket, and recipes for homemade scalp treatments, and we went home.

CHAPTER 18
HE HELD ME

I WENT TO BED as soon as I got home and woke up feeling like complete garbage—like the flu, but worse. I felt woozy, heavy, and nauseous, as if I could feel the strange, sickly resonance of each vibrating cell in my body.

I got out of bed and walked down the hallway, past our home office, where Jonathan had already started work for the day. Seeing me pass by, he followed me into the living room.

"Good morning, my love," he said cheerfully. "Can I get you anything? Water? Coffee?"

"Coffee, please." I sat in my spot on Big Brown, our cat-scratched, comfy, chocolate-brown living room couch. "I need to call my mom."

I picked up my phone and hit the button to video call my mother. She picked up immediately.

"Hi, baby." Her gaze moved around the screen, analyzing my face. "You don't look so good."

"I feel like ass," I replied.

"You look pale. What are your plans for today?"

"I think I'm just going to lie here and watch TV," I said, looking up as Jonathan carried a cup of coffee across the room.

"Here you go, love." He handed me my coffee mug, and I took a sip.

"Oh my God, this is gross." It tasted like nothing I had ever tasted before.

"What's wrong?" Mom asked.

"This coffee," I said. "I'm sorry, Jonathan. Can you take it back? It tastes disgusting. I can't drink any more." His face fell. He looked offended and defeated. He was trying to take care of me, and I just told him the coffee he made was shit. "It's not you," I backpedaled. "I think my taste buds are messed up. Like the quesadilla yesterday. It just doesn't taste right. I'm sorry."

"It's fine." He sounded dejected and waved his hand dismissively. "Here, give it to me." And he took the coffee away.

I worried about upsetting Jonathan while he was doing his best to care for me. At the same time, one of my primary senses, my taste, was completely turned upside down. I couldn't make sense of it. I didn't know why it was happening. I felt unmoored in that moment, fearing I would never regain that basic ability to enjoy food and drink again. I just hoped Jonathan could understand how this disturbance was affecting my response, and that it wasn't a personal attack on his coffee-making skills.

I spent the next two days lying on Big Brown and watching movies and TV programs that I grew up with. I didn't want to think about character arcs or complicated storylines. I just wanted to zone out to familiar programs. *The Jungle Book* and *Press Your Luck* were the perfect comfort shows. Chemo brain, brain fog from chemo, was kicking in, and my ability to concentrate was dwindling. "No whammies!" was all I could manage to focus on.

Jonathan took care of me, waiting on me hand and foot. He had always been a caring and attentive husband, but this was next-level. He sat with me while I showered, he prepared every meal whether or not I was able to eat, he cleaned the house, and he fed the cats and changed their litter. He did everything that needed to be done, all while continuing to work full-time from home, a generous allowance from his bosses and coworkers.

Being home all the time also meant he was present for every single one of my breakdowns. While "No whammies, no whammies, *stop*!" resounded from the television, I felt that familiar feeling of panic kicking in. My mouth burned, and my bones ached from the Neulasta injection. The entirety of my mouth and throat felt tingly, like the cells were wobbling and sparking with electricity. A nausea emanated from my esophagus. Between my mouth feeling like it was on fire and the gross taste of everything I tried to eat, I was on the verge of losing my damn mind.

"Jonny!" I yelled as tears welled up, the dam overflowing into a waterfall. He rushed into the living room. "I can't take it. I don't want to do it."

He sat on the nearby love seat, our knees touching, and held my hands. He didn't say much. He just sat with me.

In my sobbing fit, wailing and screaming out of illness and frustration from not being able to do anything about how I felt, my body slid off the couch and onto the floor like a toddler throwing a hissy fit. I couldn't hold myself up anymore. I just lay there, crying and screaming. Bradley and Felix peeked around the corner from the hallway, their green eyes big and filled with concern. Jonathan got down on the floor with me.

"Shhh. It's going to be OK." He petted my hair and held me.

"It's *nooooooooot*," I wailed. Strands of snot dripped from my nose, and my eyes were red and swollen. "It's *noooooooot okaaaay*." I was in full tantrum mode.

"I know." He rocked me back and forth for several minutes.

"Jonny, if I die, I want you to find someone else, OK?" I blew my nose, sniffled up my snot, and tried to catch my breath.

"That's not going to happen."

"You don't know that," I replied as we held on to each other, wrapped up like a pretzel in the middle of the floor. "It might. And I want you to be happy. You wouldn't be good alone. When you find someone, they need to treat you well. And they need to love the cats."

"OK, but that's not going to happen. I'm going to stay married to you."

I relaxed in his arms as he held me. I didn't know if I believed him. I felt like he was just saying those things to make me feel better. I felt like I was dying, And when that happened, I didn't want him to be unhappy for the rest of his life. I wanted him to be with a good person. I didn't want my death to ruin him. I didn't want him to be an old man, alone in his house with his cats, cooking himself a microwavable dinner every night. That sounded depressing. I wanted him to have a kind and loving partner to live life with, to have adventures with. I wanted him to have love again.

I checked in with my mom daily as my body felt worse and worse. There's something comforting about talking to your mom when you don't feel well. It was difficult with her being across the country, only available through phone calls and video chat. Even so, I tried to keep the conversation on my physical symptoms rather than my mental and emotional state. For some reason, I felt the responsibility to stay positive for the people outside of our home, especially my parents. I didn't want them to worry. My mom saw straight through my facade, though, as mothers typically do.

"You're not looking good," she said. "I'm going to see if I can get the COVID vaccine and come out earlier."

We had planned for her to visit toward the end of chemo, closer to the fifth infusion. Dr. B mentioned that chemo was cumulative, so symptoms got worse and more intense with each round. I thought Jonathan and I could manage by ourselves at the beginning and would need help closer to the end.

"OK," I agreed. I didn't know what to expect with chemotherapy, but feeling poisoned from the inside out wasn't it. Feeling my organs getting weaker and weaker wasn't it. And I wasn't about to reject Mom's offer to move in sooner.

The third day after chemo, I woke up feeling the worst I had felt. Feeling the worst on the third and fourth days after infusions would become a pattern. My scalp started to itch and tingle, like tiny bugs nibbling on each follicle. It was a disturbing sensation. I noticed some strands of hair on the satin pillowcase that I bought specifically with baldness in mind. I wanted a soft, silky comfort on my scalp.

"Today's the day," I told Jonathan. "I want to shave my head today."

CHAPTER 19
SHAVING MY HEAD

ONE BENEFIT OF hair salons and barbershops being closed during the pandemic was that I became the proud owner of a hair clipper set. I watched YouTube videos and cut Jonathan's hair into a mid-fade, his military hairstyle of choice. I had gotten comfortable with using the clippers.

"Where are the clippers?" Jonathan asked.

"Where they always are," I said, frustrated that my husband didn't seem to remember where anything in the house was kept. The filter between my brain and mouth took a back seat to the urgency I felt to get the prickly hair off my head. I needed to shave my head *now*. I needed to be rid of this bug follicle feeling *now*.

"Never mind. I'll get them myself." I climbed the stairs and found myself on the second floor for the first time since dismantling my Reiki studio and relocating her parts to the cold, dark basement. I let the sadness of that run through me as I retrieved the clippers and shears from the bathroom drawer. Stairs were a much more difficult task than before my first chemo session. I became winded, and my legs felt like they had bricks attached to them. My body felt beaten.

"I would have gotten them," Jonathan said when I returned. "Please don't do that again."

"OK, I'm sorry." I gathered the necessary tools needed to shave my head: hair ties, a towel, a mirror, a ruler, and a gallon-sized plastic storage bag.

"Why do you need a storage bag and ruler?" he asked.

"Because I'm going to donate my hair and need to measure it," I replied. I figured if I was going to lose my hair anyway, I should make good use of it. I was almost certain I had enough to donate as long as I cut as close to my scalp as possible.

In years past, I had made a routine of growing my hair throughout the year and cutting it short every summer, donating as many inches as I could. It may seem like a good deed, but in reality, I was just too frugal to pay for regular haircuts.

Because I let go of my hair every year, I didn't feel attached to it the way a lot of people do. I didn't feel like it defined my identity or my femininity. It was just hair. Or so I thought.

I sat down in a dining room chair, an old towel draped across my shoulders. I sectioned my hair into six pieces, making three ponytails on each side of my head. My preferred charity to donate hair to was Children With Hair Loss because they only required eight inches of hair. If I sectioned my hair strategically, I could get a closer cut without any weird angles or wasted length. I was in the middle of hair-growing season, so my hair hadn't reached its ideal length yet. I'd be cutting it close (pun totally intended).

"Can you take pictures of this?" I asked Jonathan. "I don't want to forget this moment. It's a big deal." He began taking pictures with his phone.

I picked up the shears and extended one of the ponytails. With the shears above the hair tie, I began to hack away at my hair. I could hear the crunch of each cut until the hair released. I looked in the mirror. I looked like Cynthia, Angelica's doll from *Rugrats*. *My God*, I thought. *What have I done?*

I looked up to Jonathan for reassurance. Instead of the comforting look I was seeking, he seemed shocked. He was still and staring at me. I had just gone for it without warning. Then I remembered that this was a big deal for him, too. Shaving your head because of cancer was a big deal. And I was over here completely disregarding anyone's feelings, including my own, chopping my hair off like it was just another task in the day. It was *not* just another task in the day.

"Oh my God," I said, emotion hitting me hard and fast. I wasn't prepared to feel those feelings until it was over. The only thing left to do was to keep going. I picked up the shears again and cut off the remaining sections.

Before checking my reflection, I laid out the pieces of hair on the table and lined up the ruler. They were each nine inches long. My hair could be donated. Knowing that it would go toward making a wig for a child with hair loss made my heart feel better. There was a greater purpose to my loss.

I put the smallest safety guard on the clippers and attempted to shave a path down the center of my head like a reverse Mohawk. I ran into a literal bump in the road when the clipper hit an indentation on the crown of my scalp. I've always had a slight dip in my head topography and often blamed it on my cousin throwing me into a ceiling fan when I was a baby. (It wasn't intentional. Or so he said.) Regardless of how it happened, the dip was there, and the clippers struggled.

"Would you like me to help?" Jonathan saw me having a hard

time. "I used to cut my roommate's hair in college for ROTC." I think this made him an expert in buzz cuts, so I agreed.

In one of the most compassionate acts he would ever do for me, Jonathan finished shaving my head. Hairs flew, glittering in the sunbeams shining through the window, and pieces fell to the wooden floor below. When I reached up to feel my fresh do as I looked in the mirror for the first time at a "new" version of myself, a lump formed in my throat. Emotion overtook me. *Will I ever look the same again?*

That hair represented the old me, the pre-cancer me. The me who didn't know so much suffering. The me who didn't know this kind of suffering was even possible. It was my naivety. It was my femininity and my womanhood. That morning was the last time I'd ever appear like the woman I was before, with long hair and boobs at the same time. Those things didn't make me a woman, but they were part of the woman I was and how she presented herself to the world. And now the hair was gone. The first piece was gone.

I carried myself to the bathroom to take a shower, washing away the bits of hair that stuck to my skin. I stood in the stream of hot water and cried as my tears escaped down the drain.

Jonathan swept up the hair from the dining room floor so I wouldn't see it when I returned.

CHAPTER 20
RAINBOW CHARTS

SOME PEOPLE ARE TERRIBLE in crisis situations, frozen and panicked, not knowing what to do. A smaller portion of the population is good in a crisis. These are the "run toward the fire" type of people. My mother is one of the latter. One of my earliest memories is being on a Disney vacation when I was three years old and our hotel catching on fire. People were leaning out their windows, asking vacationers on the sidewalk what was going on. The fire raged from the panes directly below. My mom grabbed her purse and the plane tickets. Then she grabbed me, and she ran. We were the first ones out of the building.

I, however, struggle in difficult situations. When I have a common cold, I am convinced it will last until my dying day. Every hangnail is a splintered plank through my finger. While I'm curled up in a ball, catastrophizing, my mother is rolling out the map, creating battle plans.

When I began chemo, some days were better than others. Some hours were better than others. Mornings were the best time of day. If I had a full night of sleep, I would wake up feeling decent. I didn't have enough energy to run a marathon, but it was enough energy to focus and feel a sense of positivity. As the day went on, that energy quickly faded.

The phrase "one day at a time" gets thrown around by people who want to be helpful. I, too, am guilty of saying this. It's a genuine sentiment, but what happens when a whole day seems like too much? I could barely think about the next thirty minutes, let alone ten hours from now. It may as well have not existed. It made no difference to me.

I learned to take each day hour by hour, sometimes minute by minute. Focusing on what was right in front of me did not come easily. I often became overwhelmed by the big picture. When each day felt like five years, how was I supposed to get through the next five months of chemo? How was I supposed to get through the next year, through surgery and radiation? It felt like this nightmare would never end.

Mom, with her stellar crisis management skills, could think of a way to get through to the other side of anything, whether it was a burning building or an afternoon after a rough bout of chemo.

When it became apparent that the issue of time and getting through it was going to be a major problem, she suggested making color-coded calendars, organized not by month but by infusion periods. Each period was three weeks, and I was scheduled for six TCHP infusions.

On a video call soon after I shaved my head and was having a "this will never end" meltdown, Mom grabbed a piece of paper and drew an example of what one of the charts would look like. It had three rows of seven-day weeks, each starting with Tuesday, the day of the week I received chemo, and boxed out like a traditional calendar. Each chart was assigned a color, in rainbow order. The first chart was red, the next was orange, then yellow, green, blue, and purple.

"As you move to the next chart, to the next infusion cycle, the color will change, and you'll feel progress as you move through the rainbow," Mom explained. "You can write down your symptoms or notes for the day in each square."

My mom has a lot of great ideas, but this was by far one of her best. I kept track of my daily symptoms in each square, which helped me see patterns from infusion to infusion.

Nauseous? *That lasted one week last time.*

Can't taste? *Your taste buds woke up on day twelve after the last infusion.*

Diarrhea? *You have to wait for week three for that to end, babe.*

I can say without question that using this method to notice patterns and progress kept me from losing my mind. It's not like it wasn't hard, though. It was hard. Every day was hard. But having written evidence that this feeling wouldn't last forever helped me get through each day. Tomorrow would be better. And the day after that would be even better.

	Tuesday	Wednesday	Thursday	Friday	Saturday	Sunday	Monday
Week 1							
Week 2							
Week 3							

CHAPTER 21
PORT FAIL

THE INCISION where my port was inserted should have been healing by now. I didn't know what that was supposed to look like since I'd never had a port before. But I was pretty sure what was happening wasn't it. As the days went on, the incision formed a large scab over it. Mom always said that scabs are God's Band-Aid, so I let it be. I didn't want to disturb my skin from healing underneath. I was careful when I bathed, and I was cautious when I changed my clothes. But nothing could have prepared me for what was to become of the port scab.

As it started falling off, it was obvious that the corner of the incision wasn't healing. That's what happens when your immune system is low—it doesn't do its job when there's a job to be done. It had been weeks. I had already received my second round of chemo. The infusion nurse, who disappointingly wasn't Jackie, pointed out that my incision wasn't looking as it should.

Concerned, I called my friend Angela, the same Angela who had sent me the fluffy pink blanket I took to my first chemo infusion. She was a nurse practitioner, and her sister was an oncology nurse.

"Send me a picture," she said. "I'll send it to my sister and see what she thinks." So I did. I had hoped she would say it looked fine, and everything was fine. But that's not what happened.

"My sister said to keep an eye on it. If it changes at all, call the on-call surgeon and let them know right away."

A few years earlier, I had bought a stool for the shower. It wasn't a nice teak stool you see in photos of aesthetic bathroom remodels. I bought an aluminum stool with a white plastic seat and cornflower-blue rubber feet. It was positively geriatric-looking. I needed something to rest my foot on as I shaved my legs, and I wanted something easy to clean that wouldn't mold. It may have been ugly, but it came in handy while bathing during chemo.

As I was preparing to shower one day, Jonathan helped me undress and take off the wound dressing over my port incision scab. The gauze was slightly dry and snagged the scab. It loosened. *Oh no*, I thought. My intuition told me that it was about to come off, and I'd see the reality of what was underneath.

In the shower, sitting on my ugly old-lady stool, I let the water hit my shoulders and run down my torso. A bead of water slipped under the scab, providing just enough pressure for it to pop off. I jumped up so fast.

"What's wrong?" Jonathan appeared like a magic act at the shower door.

"My scab fell off. I think it's bad." I turned the water off and stepped out of the shower.

I was scared to look down, so Jonathan peered at my chest first. "Hmm. That's definitely a thing."

I mustered the courage to look down. There was a hole in my chest, but the angle was such that I couldn't see into it. "Take a picture," I said. "I want to see what it looks like."

"It looks like a hole. And I'm not sure, but I think I can see your port."

I looked at the photo and was shocked. Not only is it entirely unnatural to look into your own body like that, but inside my chest hole was a piece of purple rubber. Being color-blind, Jonathan was unable to see the purple color.

"Yeah, that's not good," I said. "I'll need to call the on-call surgeon. I wonder how this will go since I'm supposed to have my third chemo tomorrow."

CHAPTER 22

MOM COMES TO TOWN

LATER THAT DAY, Jonathan and I headed to the airport to pick up my mom. I was no longer able to keep up with cooking or taking care of the house. I was in a constant daze, and my mental health was struggling from feeling poisoned and sick all the time. Not only was my mom going to take care of me, but she also planned to help Jonathan with household tasks. She is an impeccable housekeeper. When I was growing up, our home was always spotless despite three small children and pets running around making a constant mess.

Mom had bought a one-way ticket with no plans on when she would leave. She planned to stay as long as necessary and would cross the going-home bridge when it came.

It was a warm day for early April, and it felt good to get out of the house. I had on my black beanie to cover my bald head and a black swing dress. I had been gravitating toward wearing black lately. Maybe it was because it was easier not to think about coordinating clothes. Maybe it was because I wasn't feeling cheery enough to wear colors.

The airport was bustling at four in the afternoon, and Jonathan found the baggage carousel where Mom's bags would spit out. Thankfully, it was at the end of the terminal near the chairs that lined the floor-to-ceiling window. I sat while we waited.

Then I saw her. She came around the corner, holding her Vera Bradley craft bag, and her eyes were already red. We saw each other, and she started running toward me. I stood up only for her to halt right in front of me to prevent knocking me over. She gave me the gentlest yet tightest hug imaginable. She sobbed into my ear, and I realized that it was the first time she had seen me sick and bald in person.

"It's OK," I said as we embraced. "You don't have to cry. It's OK."

"I'm so glad I'm here," she wept. "I came as soon as I could."

After letting go, she wrapped her arms around Jonathan. I offered to pull one of her bags as it came off the carousel, but she wouldn't let me. It wasn't big, just carry-on size. Mom didn't see the need to bring everything she owned. Just the necessities were good enough.

As we walked to the car, I told her about my port failing and the hole in my chest. The drama had unfolded while she was in the sky. "I'll have an emergency surgery tomorrow to fix it," I told her. "So my next chemo will be postponed until Wednesday."

A concerned expression covered her face. "Will that delay affect your treatment negatively?" she asked. I told her it wouldn't, but she didn't seem convinced.

We arrived home, and Jonathan showed her the room where she'd be staying. They carried her two carry-on bags to the second floor, and I went to change into leggings and a T-shirt. I also wanted to take my beanie off and let my scalp breathe.

We met back up in the living room for a "nuffer cup" after she settled in. At home in Pennsylvania, we'd often sit together in the afternoon for a cup of hot tea. Conversation flowing, we'd ask if the other person wanted another cup, which eventually morphed into "nuffer cup."

Jonathan filled the kettle, and Mom sat on the love seat, Big Brown's little sister, after her long travel day. I walked around the corner into the room, and Mom's face looked shocked, as if her body had internally gasped at my sight. It was the first time she'd seen me bald in person. Reality was setting in for her. Seeing me with a beanie on was one thing. It wasn't much different from wearing a hat or a headscarf, something I did regularly when I had hair. But seeing her child bald for the first time in person was something she couldn't have prepared herself for, no matter how hard she tried. And I had a hard time watching her attempt to hide her emotions from me. I had done everything I could to protect my parents from worrying, but I could no longer do that now that Mom was here. She would be present for everything from this point forward—every medication dose, every breakdown, every tear. I was grateful for her presence.

CHAPTER 23
LIKE A HOLE IN MY CHEST

THE DAY AFTER Mom moved in, Jonathan took me to the hospital to have my port replaced. The surgeon was perplexed about why it hadn't healed properly and determined that the massive doses of chemotherapy were to blame. He promised to triple-stitch the new port into place to prevent the incision from opening again.

"What about the old port location?" I asked. "Will you stitch that up too?"

"No," he said. "We don't want to close in any bacteria that might have gotten in, so we're going to leave it open, and you guys will have to pack it until it heals. The nurse will give you the wound packing instructions."

Wound packing. That's just great. I wasn't scared of the surgery, but the idea of packing a one-inch wound hole twice a day made my skin crawl.

I opted for twilight drugs over general anesthesia this time around because that meant being able to leave the clinic sooner. Fortunately, unlike my friend, I didn't remember anything from the procedure, and I was home by lunchtime.

That evening, when it was time to change the dressing, Jonathan, my mom, and I all crammed into our tiny bathroom. Jonathan took the lead. He removed the tape and outer layer of gauze from my chest and paused to gauge the situation. As I sat on the closed toilet lid, Mom bent over to evaluate what we were dealing with. She'd dealt with all sorts of wounds and boo-boos from us kids. She had seen heads gashed open and had tweezed bark from my five-year-old gums after I'd run into a tree while laughing during a game of tag. Let's just say that Grace wasn't my middle name. In fact, my childhood nickname was Boo-Boo Girl, fitting for my clumsy and aloof ways.

"You ready?" Jonathan asked as he prepared to remove the packing from the hole where the old port once sat.

"Yup." I braced for the worst, not knowing what to expect.

Jonathan slowly pulled out the saline-soaked gauze. It seemed never-ending. It just kept coming and coming until eventually about a foot of gauze lay on the bathroom counter.

"Wow," he said. "That's a thing."

My mom stared at my chest, mouth agape. I didn't know what to think but felt scared. "How big is the hole?" I asked.

"About the size of a quarter," Mom answered. "It's pretty deep. Do you want to see it?" It was too high on my chest for me to look down and view, so she held up a mirror. I took one glance and looked away. It was much bigger than I had anticipated.

The clinic had sent us home with a bunch of sterile saline to soak the fresh gauze in before stuffing it into my wound. If dry, it would stick to the tissue when it was time to pull it out and be counterproductive to healing. Jonathan drenched the gauze in saline and gently filled the hole. I sat still with my eyes closed and took deep breaths. The sensation wasn't painful but was unnatural and disturbing. Mom stood in the background, humming Disney melodies. This coping mechanism was meant to calm her down just as much as it was to calm me down.

They took turns packing my chest every morning and night for the next three months.

CHAPTER 24
DOVE AND OTHER JOYS

ALL I WANTED to do was sit on the couch and rot. I wanted to watch comfort shows while Bradley purred on my lap. I didn't want to do anything productive, and I definitely didn't want to do anything active while feeling so terrible. But Mom wasn't having it.

"I don't think it's good for you to sit around all day," she said. "I think we should get out of the house at least once a day."

"Get out of the house?" I said, exasperated. "This chemo has me feeling like I'm going to poop my pants at any second. I'm not leaving the house." One of the chemotherapy drugs wasn't nicknamed Poopy Perjeta for nothing.

"We don't have to go far. Even if we just sit on the front porch. It'll be good to get some sun on your face."

As much as I hate to admit it, Mom is usually right. And she was right. On days when I felt like smashed trash, usually at the beginning of each chemo cycle, sitting on the porch was as much as I could tolerate. Being more than thirty seconds from the nearest bathroom was a no-go.

Sitting on the front steps, sun on my face and breeze on my scalp, was a welcome intermission to the day. Getting off the couch was tough. Sitting down on the concrete step was difficult without support, but once I got into place, it felt nice. It felt like I was part of the world again. The sound of cars on the next road over, the joyous laughter of kids riding their bikes down the sidewalk, the smell of freshly cut grass from a few houses over all felt, dare I say, normal. I could take my mind off my sickness and suffering, at least for the moment.

My mother is a bird whisperer. At her house, she sits on her front porch watching the hummingbirds and robins make their home in her yard. Sometimes the hummingbirds will pause in front of her, flapping their speedy wings while hovering in place, as if to thank her for the sugar water she puts out for them every few days. Nature and her creatures are Mom's forte. I wasn't surprised when she took note of the birds in my neighborhood while we soaked up Utah's spring sunrays.

"There's this dove that keeps flying to your front tree," she said as she got up to investigate the tree in question. "Emily, come here. This is incredible."

I grabbed the railing and hoisted myself up. My leg strength was worsening by the day. For someone who used to have thick, muscular thighs and a booty to match, you wouldn't know it. That's how weak I was becoming. I slowly shuffled along the sidewalk, making my way to the tree Mom was looking at. The leaves had recently sprouted and were becoming thicker, making it tricky to see what she was looking at.

"Look between these branches." She pointed through the leaves to something. "She's sitting in a nest. Shhh. Don't make too much noise and scare her." I tilted my head to see where she was pointing, and I saw her. "We should name her."

"What should we name her?" I asked.

"Dove," Mom replied.

From that day forward, I checked on Dove every day. When she wasn't in her nest, I could see there were eggs she was brooding. It was springtime after all, and I wondered if they'd hatch soon. Sometimes when I checked on her, there was a second dove in the nest.

"I think that's her husband," I told Mom. "His name is Doveward." Dove and Doveward sitting in a tree. I did my best not to bother them and their growing family. I just quickly glanced each day to make sure they were OK. It gave me something to look forward to. Something outside of myself.

One day after checking on Dove, I thought the urge to go was manageable. Out of the three-week chemo cycle, I was only nervous about pooping myself during the second week, after the Perjeta set into my system. It was the tail end of Poop Week, and I felt brave enough to venture farther away from home with a walk around the block.

"Let's give it a try," Mom said. "If you can't make it, we can always turn back." She went inside to grab our shoes, and off we went, moving as slow as molasses. We'd only made it to the sidewalk in front of my next-door neighbor's house when I stopped in my tracks.

"Oh no," I said with urgency in my voice.

"What's wrong?" Mom said in a panicked breath, grabbing my arm, fearful that I might fall.

"I'm fine," I replied, slightly annoyed. "But I need to go back. Right now." I hoped she caught my drift. I didn't want to say out loud that I was about to shit myself for fear that the neighbor's doorbell camera would pick it up. My neighbor was cool, and we were friendly, but we weren't at that level of friendship.

I didn't want her to know about my sudden diarrhea, and I certainly didn't want it to be recorded for anyone to look back on and laugh at my misfortune for eternity. We turned around, and I scurried the fifty feet back to my front door, making it inside and to the toilet in the nick of time. It was a close call, but I didn't poop my pants.

A few days later, when Poop Week had finally passed, I gained more confidence to explore farther away from home, this time a walk around the neighborhood. My bowels were in good order, and I felt like my legs could handle a longer walk.

Mom stayed close by my side as we walked through the neighborhood, through the nearby park, and back to the house.

"Do you want to try to go a little farther?" she asked. I was up for it, and the weather was cooperating, so why not? We crossed the street that separated our neighborhood from the nearby townhouse community. I had never walked through that area. I hoped we wouldn't get lost, as I was known to be navigationally challenged. One time, I missed the exit while returning home and didn't notice until an hour later. Even though the townhouses were adjacent to our own neighborhood, I wouldn't put it past myself to get lost for hours. Nevertheless, we pressed on, making note of where the mountains were in the distance in relation to my house. The Wasatch Mountains were always a good navigational guide in the Salt Lake Valley.

As we weaved through the townhouses and the curving sidewalks that separated them, I was surprised by all the beauty that was right under my nose. I hadn't noticed it before, hadn't known it was all there. Beautiful flower beds. Bumblebees working hard to pollinate adjacent plants. A community vegetable garden. Each time we passed the garden, Mom would point out the different vegetables and when they should be planted and harvested.

Walking home, we passed an electrical box hidden by a rosebush planted next to it. The buds were still closed, but with the warming weather, they would bloom any day. As with the vegetable garden, each time we passed, we'd take note of the roses' blooming progress.

Over the next few months, as chemo treatment progressed, Mom and I continued walking this path on good days. The vegetable plants yielded tomatoes, peppers, and lettuce. The rosebush bloomed in her full raspberry-red glory. Mom was right. By getting out into the world with the warmth of the sun and the sweet smell of nature, I was able to gain more hope for what my world could look like after cancer.

"You have to keep your spirits up," she said. "You have to try."

Dove's eggs never hatched that summer.

CHAPTER 25
A NEW HOBBY

THE INTERNET is a terrifying place full of scary statistics and stories of suffering. It's also a supportive place to find a community of people with similar experiences.

When I was diagnosed, I had joined several cancer-related social media groups, each supporting different demographics, including young breast cancer survivors, breast cancer patients who chose to go flat instead of having reconstruction, and IBC survivors.

One day, as I was lying on the couch and feeling like crap, I read a post from someone who had asked, "How do you guys keep your mind from obsessing during chemo?" The comments were full of suggestions, but the most common advice was to start a new hobby.

Start a new hobby? I'm sorry, but I'm having my body pumped full of poison. I can barely make it to the toilet on time, and you expect me to take up painting? You must be out of your damn mind. My body hurt, my brain was too foggy to think, and my only focus was not pooping my pants. I couldn't understand how someone could even *consider* suggesting that a dying person take on a new hobby.

So I took up cross-stitch.

On a day when I had just enough energy to leave the house and wasn't worried about having diarrhea in public, Mom and I went to a nearby craft store. She was an avid crocheter and cross-stitcher. She'd taught me a few skills over the years, but I never had the patience for cross-stitch. We ventured down the stitching aisle as she looked for a tool she needed. While I was waiting for her, I spotted the cross-stitch kits, complete with everything necessary to complete a project.

"Look at this one," I said. "I want to make this for my friend." It was a colorful image of flowering cacti with bright greens and pinks. It was the first time I had been drawn to bright colors in a while. "Can you teach me to cross-stitch?" I asked.

"Yes, of course," Mom said excitedly as I handed her the kit. "This might be really good for your fingers, too. It'll get the blood flowing." Chemo was giving me a nasty case of neuropathy in my fingers, causing the tips to feel numb, yet stabbed by pins and needles at the same time. The doctor had suggested moving my fingers to keep blood circulating.

We bought the kit and took it home. As we sat in our usual places on the couch, Mom showed me how to begin stitching, how to make stitches look consistent, and how to tie off a completed section.

In the days and weeks that followed, I became obsessed with stitching. I stitched all day, every day, while *Schitt's Creek*, another comfort show that I was watching for the second time through, ran in the background.

I finished the cactus project in just a few weeks and soon wanted to do more. Making a gift for someone else helped keep my focus off myself and my suffering. The lesson here is that if you ever feel like you're slowly being poisoned and dying, learn a new hobby.

CHAPTER 26
CIRCLES OF SUPPORT

EVERY THIRD TUESDAY, there I was again, sitting in the chemo chair at the infusion center. I preferred the spot in front of the floor-to-ceiling window overlooking the beautiful Wasatch Mountains and a Red Lobster. Nothing says "You got this!" like looking at the roof of a seafood restaurant for eight hours straight.

The nurse had just set up one of my IV bags when Lilly, my oncology team's licensed clinical social worker, came in. I was always excited to see Lilly when she stopped by. She was a breath of fresh air in a sterile, clinical environment.

"Hey guys! Sorry I'm late. There was a meeting that ran over."

"It's totally OK," I said. "We're here all day." She chuckled at my lame attempt at a joke.

I felt like Lilly understood me. Jonathan and I had both confided in her about all the feelings we were having through this process. She always had the perfect advice and insight. It's like she worked exclusively with cancer patients or something. Because she did.

"So what's going on?" she asked as she leaned against the wall. "How's everything going? Is there anything I can help with today?"

Jonathan expressed concerns about the best ways to support me during treatment. I was more concerned about how to support those around me. I knew that this process and seeing me suffer was difficult for those I was closest to. I told Lilly my thoughts on this.

"Have you ever heard of circles of support or Ring Theory?" she asked me.

"No. What's that?"

"It's a theory that explains how we receive support from the people around us," she explained. "Ring Theory started with a psychologist named Susan Silk. Picture a bull's-eye of circles, like on a dartboard." She formed her hands in the shape of a circle. "You're in the middle. The circles revolve around you and are here to support you. On the second tier of circles are the people who are closest to you, the people who live with you, like Jonathan and your mom. On the next tier are people you love, but aren't your closest people. This would be family or close friends. Next are friends and co-workers, then acquaintances, then strangers." She moved her hands farther outward with each tier mentioned.

OK, what does this have to do with me right now? I wondered.

"The idea surrounding the circles of support is that people receive support from the outer tiers of the circle and give support to the inner tiers of the circle. Support inward, and vent outward. Since you're the one going through this really hard thing, you're not meant to give support to the outer tiers. Jonathan and your mom are meant to receive support from *their* outer tiers, people like your dad or Jonathan's parents. And they in turn receive support from their outer tiers. They all give support inward, and ultimately to you as the person in the center. Your only job is healing, not worrying about supporting those around you."

"Wow," I said. "That's really hard."

"It is for a lot of people," she said. "But it allows you to focus on the only thing you need to worry about, which is healing. We don't want you to spend energy on anything else. You need to allow Jonathan's and your mom's circles of support to support them. That's not for you to worry about right now."

As the person who was always taking care of those around me, this was a challenging concept. I had to learn to trust people in the outer circles—my dad, Laura, and Jonathan's parents—to care for Jonathan and my mom.

As difficult as trusting sometimes is, this concept made sense to me. Of course, I would always worry about how they were holding up or handling everything we were going through. But I made a promise to both Lilly and myself that I would focus solely on getting better.

The Circles of Support

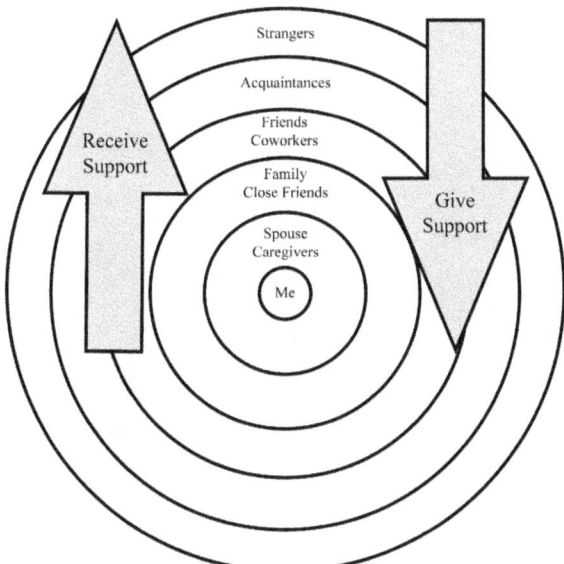

CHAPTER 27
WIG

AS MOM FELT increasingly comfortable taking care of me during the day and managing my medication regimen, Jonathan slowly transitioned to going back into the office. Being around people again provided a huge benefit to his mental health. Doing normal things, like the simple routine of going to work, was good for his spirit.

In May, with less than a month of my systemic chemo, TCHP, remaining, Jonathan was going to be promoted. He scheduled the ceremony for the third week of my chemo cycle so I could be there. I'd been present for every major event in his military career to date, and I didn't want to miss it.

Although everyone he worked with knew that I had cancer, I was still self-conscious of my bald head. When my hair fell out, I was left with sporadic single hairs on random parts of my scalp. I hadn't yet thought to just shave them off, and I felt like Babyface, the mutant toy made of a doll's head and Erector set crab legs from Sid's bedroom in *Toy Story*.

My oncologist prescribed a wig when I was concerned about losing my hair. I didn't know doctors could write a prescription for a wig, but it turns out they can. I had chosen one that looked similar to my natural hairstyle and decided to wear it to Jonathan's promotion to look as normal as possible in photos.

Mom carried a kitchen chair to my bedroom. I sat as she helped put on my wig. Although the lady at the wig store taught me how to put it on, I had never done it on my own before and had no idea what I was doing.

"How do you want me to style it?" Mom asked, also not knowing anything about wigs.

"Just like how I used to do my hair. It's a good wig, so you can use hot tools if you need to." My insurance hadn't yet reimbursed me, and I had spent way too much money on a high-quality wig simply so I could style it with a straightener or curling iron.

The wig was already wavy like my natural hair, so she didn't use hot tools, but she did use bobby pins to place the waves so they framed my face. She attempted a half-up, half-down hairdo.

"Mom, I look like someone from *Little House on the Prairie*."

"What? You do not. I think it looks nice."

"Can you try to fix it?" I asked. "So it's not so old-fashioned? We should have practiced before today."

She carefully pulled bobby pins out of the wig, one by one. On one pull of a pin, the wig slipped across my scalp, off the back of my head, and onto the floor as if in slow motion. Mom froze, not sure what to do. I could tell she was stifling a smile but didn't want me to feel embarrassed.

I cracked up laughing. Embracing humor through the weird stuff gets you through the tough stuff. Mom started laughing, too.

She restyled the wig until I accepted how it looked. I put on some light makeup and adorned the three eyelashes I had left with mascara. We made our way to the military base for Jonathan's promotion.

Everyone was friendly to both Mom and me, but my head itched the entire time. I just wanted to rip that wig off my head. It was so uncomfortable.

I saw a few photos of the promotion ceremony after we got home and thought I looked ridiculous wearing fake hair. I tried to reflect on why I cared so much about looking like my old self for this event. Being bald was my reality. This was how it was. Why was I trying to pretend that it wasn't? Nobody cared that I was bald, especially not our military family. They were just glad I could be there, no matter what I looked like.

After seeing those photos, I decided to embrace my baldness. It was authentic to who I was in that moment, authentic to what I was going through.

I never wore that expensive, itchy wig again.

CHAPTER 28
THERAPY CATS

ONE DAY AFTER WORK, Jonathan's coworker Lauren asked him if I'd like to meet her therapy cat.

"What's a therapy cat?" I asked him. I'd had cats my whole life and had never heard of this. I knew about service dogs and emotional support animals, but never a therapy cat.

"He's just a big cuddly cat," he guessed. "I'm not really sure."

Big cuddly cat? Say less. "Yes! I want to meet her cat!"

I had only met Lauren once at a large family-friendly work event, and she seemed nice. She had recently gotten a Ragdoll kitten named Mochi. Her previous Ragdoll, Indy, was a therapy cat, but had sadly passed away. She would take Indy to nursing homes and college campuses (during finals week) to relieve residents' and students' stress. Everyone loved Indy.

Mochi was still young and in training. Lauren thought it might be a good opportunity for him to work with someone who had cancer. I met Lauren and Mochi at a nearby park, and when I walked toward the picnic table I saw the most beautiful fluffy, blue-eyed white-and-brown cat I'd ever seen. Mochi greeted me with sniffs, and I was soon holding him in my arms like a baby. With all the stress of cancer, I could feel my cortisol lowering as I held this big ball of floof. I cuddled Mochi for about an hour while Jonathan, Lauren, and I chatted under the gazebo.

"I can bring him to your house sometime if you're open to it," Lauren offered.

"I would love that," I said. "But we have two other cats. Would he be OK with that? Felix is friendly, and Bradley would probably hide under a bed."

"If you're OK with it, I'm good with it," she assured me. "It might be a good thing for him to practice being around other animals besides his siblings."

A few weeks later, Lauren brought Mochi to the house. Felix swiftly greeted them at the door. His nickname is Friendly Felix for a reason. He loves making new friends. He loves other cats, but he doesn't know how to respect their personal space. Felix doesn't like boundaries.

Lauren and I sat on the couch while Mochi became comfortable with his surroundings. Jonathan attempted to distract Felix in the bedroom. I picked Mochi up and held him in my arms while he purred. A calmness entered my body just as it did in the park.

I enjoyed spending time with Lauren. She was one of the few people who didn't treat me like I was sick. She didn't look at me with pity. She treated me like a normal person, like she would treat anyone else. We talked about things going on in our lives, just like any pair of friends would do.

"Do you want to see how he does with Felix?" Lauren asked.

"OK. He might get excited and overwhelm Mochi."

"We can try and see how it goes," she said. It was her first time meeting Felix, and I wasn't sure she knew what Mochi was about to get himself into.

Jonathan went to the bedroom and brought Felix out. They sniffed each other's noses and became fast friends. That is, until

Felix got "the look" in his eyes. The look says, *You're my best friend, and I want to be right next to you forever and ever.*

An overwhelmed Mochi took refuge under the couch. Felix sat at the edge, as if to say, *Don't worry, friend. I'm waiting right here for you to come out.* As Lauren extracted Mochi from beneath the couch to take him home, Mochi had a look of terror in his eyes.

Not giving up, Mochi came over for practice therapy sessions a few more times, but Lauren decided that he wasn't cut out to be a therapy cat. I blame it on Felix's aggressive friendship. I felt awful that Felix caused him to fail therapy cat training.

Thankfully, I didn't have the same effect on Lauren. We've remained good friends, and I enjoy visiting Mochi at their home. His cuddles are still as stress-reducing as ever, and I highly recommend a therapy cat's services to anyone.

CHAPTER 29

NOT DOING THIS ANYMORE

THE FARTHER ALONG I got through TCHP, systemic chemo, the worse I felt. That was to be expected given that chemo is cumulative and builds up in the system over time. I was three months into treatment and reminded myself that it was normal to feel increasingly worse.

My walks with Mom became shorter and less frequent. Some days, I could make it only to the rosebush on the next block. I didn't check on Dove as often. Getting up and moving was harder. Some days I showered, and some days I didn't. The act of taking off my clothes and washing my scalp and skin was exhausting. And since chemo killed just about everything in my body, I didn't have skin bacteria to create body odor. Hygiene wasn't my top priority, but I knew I had to bathe, so this task was saved for every other day. I didn't care. I had very few cares anymore.

My mouth tingled and burned. Everything tasted terrible. The only thing I could taste normally was cottage cheese, an odd thing to crave when I constantly felt like I might vomit. I was surprised that I never actually puked through my entire chemo experience. It wasn't easy, and I certainly wanted to. I even tried to vomit once, thinking it would make me feel better. But the nurse's words echoed in the back of my mind: *If you puke, you'll get dehydrated and end up in the hospital. So please try your very best not to puke.* So I stopped.

Chemo brain, the brain fog that accompanies chemotherapy, was in full effect. I used to have a type A personality with a sharp mind. I regularly anticipated what others needed before they asked. I was reliable, detail-oriented, and on top of everything. Not anymore. My memory was shit, and I often didn't remember to thank friends when they sent me blankets. It was so unlike me, but my brain was fried.

My muscles were weak, and my bones hurt. Simply walking from the bedroom to the couch was challenging. My legs felt like Jell-O, and I frequently lost my balance, grabbing on to a nearby person or piece of furniture for support.

"I think you should think about getting a wheelchair," Mom said one day as I returned to the couch from the bathroom, taking extreme care with every step.

"Wheelchair? No. Absolutely not. I'm not getting a wheelchair." I was firm.

"I think it might help," she insisted. "I'm so worried about you falling and hurting yourself."

"I'm not getting a wheelchair. I don't want to look sicker than I already am."

"Would you consider a cane at least?"

"Fine," I submitted. "I'll consider a cane."

At age thirty-five, I bought my first cane. To my surprise, it helped my balance significantly. (Mom was right again. How does that always happen?) I actually liked my cane. It wasn't much to look at, not fancy at all. Black aluminum with a rubber handle, it was lightweight and easy to use. I channeled my inner Bert from

Mary Poppins, attempting to feel less disabled and more debonair. Even so, walking still zapped my daily energy, and at times, I did wish I had a wheelchair. But I felt like I had to try. I had to try to walk. I had to try to be normal, whatever normal is when you're in that situation.

My daily goal was to make it to bed each night. Once in bed, Mom would come in to give me a hug and kiss before heading up to her bedroom, like I was a child being tucked in at the end of the day. It was nostalgic and comforting, even as an adult woman. There's something about the body relaxing after a day of trying to physically survive. It's like my body was on high alert, in survival mode all day. Then once my body hit the mattress and relaxed, my mind took over. The fear and anxiety accompanied by the physical feeling of each organ being poisoned left me teetering on the edge of my thinly veiled sanity.

Many nights, especially the few nights right after an infusion, I would cry, then wail. Maybe it was the pain. Maybe it was the feeling of dying. But I felt like I couldn't physically do it anymore.

"I'm not doing it anymore," I said, sobbing and hyperventilating. "I'm not doing any more chemo."

"Yes, you are," Mom said emphatically. "You have to. You have to try." The idea of me giving up was not an option to her. I was her child, and children are not supposed to die before their parents. Her motherly response was to tell me what I was going to do. I *was* going to finish chemo, like it or not.

"Well, I'm not!" I yelled. "I'm not doing it anymore. I'm done."

Jonathan knew there was no convincing me otherwise. "OK," he said. "We can talk to the doctor about that."

I had a visit with the oncologist before every infusion to check in on how I was doing and to make sure that my blood counts were good enough to handle chemo that day. "I'm going to tell her I'm not doing this anymore."

"OK," he repeated. "We'll talk to her about that."

Chemo day eventually rolled back around, and I always found myself back in the infusion chair with the understanding that each of them would be my last.

"I'll do this next one," I said every time. "But this is my last one." I said it after my third infusion, then the fourth and fifth, until it was finally time for my sixth and final TCHP infusion, my last dose of systemic chemo, my last dose of poison being distributed to every cell in my body.

"I'll do this one," I told Mom the morning before leaving the house for the final round. "But I swear to *Gawd*, I'm not doing this again! And I mean it this time."

"OK," she said. "You don't have to do it again."

CHAPTER 30
THE SMILING STRANGER EFFECT

I MIGHT HAVE finished chemo, but I didn't ring the bell. Not yet. I still had plenty of cancer treatment left—a double mastectomy and radiation. My mastectomy was scheduled for six weeks after my last TCHP infusion. The surgeon wanted to give my immune system time to get to a better place, time for my body to heal before slicing it open. A mastectomy is a major surgery, and with any major surgery, there's always a risk of infection. My white blood cells had to be in tip-top shape to heal properly.

As I made it past the hardest weeks following the last chemo, I felt like I was floating on a cloud. The promise of not having more chemo was invigorating. I still needed a cane, but my energy was improving. My mental health was soaring. I wanted to get out and live life. The universe must have heard me because we soon received an invitation to our real estate agent's annual "family picnic." All his past clients were invited, and the event was promised to be a fun time with raffles, food trucks, and face painting. And who doesn't love face painting? Nobody, that's who. Face painting is fun for all ages.

It was drill weekend for the Air National Guard, so Jonathan had to work, but Mom and I were eager to get out of the house. I hadn't been around many people since beginning chemo because of my compromised immune system, but my health was improving by the day, and the event was outdoors with plenty of space to distance myself from others.

Something interesting happens when the side effects of cancer are visible. My bald head, pale skin, and cane left nothing to the imagination. It was clear that I was sick. When Mom and I arrived at the picnic, I stood out like a sore thumb. After being isolated for months, I was self-conscious about my appearance.

My nerves calmed down when we walked to the sign-in table and saw our real estate agent. Not long after I had announced my diagnosis, he brought a huge gorgeous orchid to the house. He was more than a guy who sold us a home. He was a good, caring person.

"Emily!" he said, greeting me with arms in the air.

"Are you vaccinated?" I asked. I was still worried about catching COVID-19.

"I am," he said. I passed my cane to my mom and gave him a big hug. It was the first time I'd hugged anyone outside of Jonathan, my mom, and my oncologist in over five months. It was nice to see a friend.

"This is my mom," I said, introducing them.

"Mom!" he exclaimed, embracing my mother with equal enthusiasm.

After catching up, we made our way to the picnic tables under a giant gazebo. I sat in the shade while Mom plated food for both of us. It was one of the first hot days of the year, and I decided to take off my beanie, revealing my bald head for the first time in public. I had shaved off the random stubbles a few days before, so it was baby-butt smooth. I knew it didn't matter, but I was nervous about what others would think of me. Every single person who passed by flashed a big smile. One family asked to sit next to us to make us feel included.

The "smiling stranger" effect lasted almost a full year until my hair grew back. Strangers smiled, opened doors for me, and struck up conversations. As the weather continued to heat up for the summer, I wore my beanie less frequently. What was I worried about? That I didn't have hair? I was sick. It was what it was. This was my body now, and I wanted to be comfortable, not sweating under a hat.

I often think back to this time and wonder what would happen if society treated everyone the way I was treated when I was bald. Although I was sometimes self-conscious, it warmed my heart to know and feel the compassion of strangers. People were kindhearted. I think about how they made me feel and how I want others to feel when they're around me.

At the risk of looking slightly unhinged, I try to smile at strangers as often as possible now. I try to show kindness to others in public. I tell people when I like their shoes or their shirt. I want people to feel good about themselves, the same way others made me feel good about myself when I didn't feel that way on my own. If everyone showed genuine empathy and compassion, the world would be a better place. We all have much more in common than we do differences.

CHAPTER 31
THE TOLL OF STRESS

IT'S NO SECRET that stress negatively impacts the body. I can't think of anything more stressful than your child or your spouse having cancer. While I was going through treatment and focused on myself, my mom and Jonathan were busy taking care of me *and* themselves. Because of the circles of support, neither expressed their fear of me dying, at least not to me. But I knew they were both feeling it. Self-care was essential for them both. It's not easy being a caregiver.

Jonathan had work to keep his mind busy, and he talked to his family often. He was able to keep his routine fairly normal. But Mom was in another state, away from her home, with me all day, every day. I was always there, looking sick and frequently crying, a constant reminder that her child might die.

Mom did her best to take care of herself. Before I woke up each morning, she would take a walk. It was a time to release stress, explore the neighborhood and plants, and become familiar with the birds, just as we did on our joint walks. My mom was never a heavy eater, but I noticed her eating less over time. She lost twenty-four pounds in three months, and her clothes had become loose on her body. Her gut was reacting to the constant state of fight-or-flight mode.

It was easy for her to hide her struggles from me. Some afternoons while I was eyeballs-deep in my cross-stitch project, she told me she needed to go upstairs and take a nap. By the time she was behind the wall and just out of sight, she'd be crying already. Instead of napping, she'd lie in bed and cry. She called my dad and would unload her burdens onto him. Her nervous system was freaking out, and her body function was suffering.

The weekend after our real estate agent's picnic, Jonathan suggested taking an adventure. He wanted to show Mom the Bonneville Salt Flats, a vast area of salt landscape in the western part of Utah. Standing on the salt flats feels like what I imagine standing on the surface of the moon feels like, surreal and otherworldly. It's something every Utah tourist should visit. We drove two hours to the rest stop off I-80, the best place to stop and take pictures, and took it all in. I could tell Mom was enjoying being in nature, witnessing this incredible landscape the universe had created.

When I shuffled into the living room, cane in hand for balance, the next morning—which was the Fourth of July, Independence Day in the USA—I noticed that Mom wasn't in her usual spot on the couch waiting for me.

"Where's Mom?" I asked Jonathan, who was making a cup of coffee in the kitchen.

"I don't know. I haven't seen her yet."

Just then, Mom stepped slowly down the stairs.

"I was up all night." She looked pale and clammy. "I'm really not feeling well. Jonathan, can you take me to the hospital?"

I thought maybe she'd caught a bug being out in society's germs and just needed to be rehydrated with fluids.

The nearest hospital was only a few minutes away. Jonathan dropped her off while I waited at home.

"They took her right back," he said when he returned. "No wait at all."

"I'm sure it'll be busier tonight after everyone blows off their fingers from fireworks," I replied. "Good thing she'll be home by then." Nearly dying was bringing out my dark sense of humor.

A short time later, my phone rang. It was Mom. She sounded loopy and drugged.

"They gave me medicine for my pain to help me calm down." Her words were slurred. *I can tell*, I thought. "The doctor wants to talk to you. I told him he could talk to my daughter."

The next voice I heard was the doctor's. He told me how they weren't sure what was going on with Mom, and they wanted to send her to the University of Utah's main hospital for more testing. Since it was a federal holiday, resources were limited at the satellite clinic. She needed to go by ambulance, and someone would call me after she arrived. He was saying this like he was reading the menu at Olive Garden. *There's soup, salad, breadsticks, and an ambulance ride.* He handed the phone back to Mom.

"I'm scared," she said. She was crying.

I felt my cortisol rising, anxiety filling my chest. Mom was always the one to take us kids to the hospital for broken bones or stitches. I'd never known my mother to be sick like this. "I know," I said. "It's going to be OK. The U is the best. Jonathan and I will be on our way once we find out where you are."

We visited Mom at the university hospital over the next three days. It was strange to see her lying in a hospital bed. I'd never seen that before, and it was upsetting. Doctors performed every test they could, but every result was normal. There was no physical explanation for her illness.

As gently as he could, the doctor explained that he thought her symptoms were due to stress, and he recommended that she go back home to Pennsylvania as soon as possible to be closer to her own medical team, where she could be monitored. I felt like he was trying to let me down easy, as if to say *I know you have cancer, but your mom can't be here to take care of you.* He had to say it because she never would.

"I'm so sorry." Mom cried into the scratchy hospital sheets. "I'm supposed to be here to take care of you. I'm supposed to help you through surgery."

"It's OK," I reassured her. I was primarily worried about her well-being, not my surgery. If I made it through chemo, I could make it through anything.

A few days after she entered the hospital, Mom was released and came back to our house. Jonathan bought her a one-way ticket back to Pennsylvania and upgraded her to first class. She deserved it.

It was time to call in the backup team.

CHAPTER 32

THE IN-LAWS ARE COMING

WE RETURNED from the airport and called my in-laws, Karen and Wayne.

"What do you need from us?" Karen asked. "What can we do to help you guys?"

"Can you come?" I asked her. "I know it's short notice. Only a couple of weeks until surgery. But I wanted to know if you'd be able to come."

Karen, a nurse practitioner, had worked in medicine for more than thirty years. If there was anyone who was equipped to help me during a major surgical recovery, it was her. Although she had offered to help from the beginning, I felt bad asking her to travel across the country at the last minute.

"Yes, of course," she said. "And Wayne will come too."

"Is he able to do that?" Jonathan asked his mom. "It's not an issue with his job?" Wayne, Jonathan's stepfather, was only a few months away from retirement and had been saving up his vacation days to cash in at the end of his career.

"I'll take my vacation days," Wayne chimed in from beyond the camera's reach. "Don't even worry about it. It's no big deal. I'll take as much time off as I can."

Aside from my mom taking three months out of her life to move in with me, this was one of the most generous offers anyone had proposed. I had a hard time asking for help. It didn't come naturally to me. The idea that someone would offer to use all their vacation time to help us was beyond me, and I was grateful. I also felt incredibly guilty, as if I were an inconvenience. I didn't want to be an inconvenience to anyone.

"As long as you're sure," I said. "Only as long as you're sure."

CHAPTER 33

BOOBS FOR SCIENCE

THE NEXT FEW WEEKS felt surreal. It was just Jonathan and me alone for the first time in months. My symptoms had improved, and I was beginning to feel life force energy reentering my body. My state of mind was improving. It's amazing how the condition of the physical body affects the mind and spirit as much as it does. I could taste food again. My mouth wasn't on fire. My bones didn't ache. I wasn't nauseous. Although I was still fatigued, I felt on top of the world. Chemo was the worst thing I had gone through, and it was over.

A few days before surgery, I received a phone call from a woman in the research department at the cancer hospital.

"I know this is short notice," she said. "As you know, your case is different from the majority of breast cancer cases. We wanted to know if you'd be willing to donate your breast tissue to the University of Utah's research department."

"Oh my God, of course," I said immediately. I didn't need to think about it. The idea of my boobs going to research to help other women with IBC gave me an instant feeling of comfort and peace. "What do I have to do?"

"Oh wow, thank you so much." She sounded surprised at my quick enthusiasm to give her my boobs. "I'm going to email you some paperwork to sign. I know it's rushed, but if you could do that by tomorrow, we'd appreciate it."

"No problem at all," I replied. "I'm happy that they'll help other people." I watched my inbox like a hawk and signed the consent paperwork as soon as it arrived.

After I agreed to donate my boobs to science, I thought about all the breast tissue that isn't donated to research. Do they just throw the boobs in the trash? Hold a funeral and bury them? What happens to other people's boobs? I didn't know. But that wasn't going to be my boobs. My boobs wouldn't be tossed in the trash or treated like toxic waste. They would be sliced up and stored in a freezer at the University of Utah. For science. For other women with IBC to have a better chance at life. And that was a good feeling.

CHAPTER 34
A LETTER TO MY BOOBS

KAREN AND WAYNE arrived the evening before my surgery, packed for a two-week stay. A trip to the airport was a welcome distraction from my nervous energy. My boobs would be amputated tomorrow.

My "showtime" wasn't until eleven o'clock in the morning, and I wasn't allowed to eat past midnight due to the anesthesia. I tried to stay up as late as possible that night so I could eat promptly at 11:59 p.m. to prevent hunger the next day. Being a breakfast eater my whole life, I knew I would be starving in the morning. I tended to become hangry if I didn't eat breakfast. Nobody wanted that, especially me.

As I lay in bed, trying to keep my eyes open, I crossed my arms and held my boobs just like I did in the shower the morning I discovered the cancer. This would be one of the last times I'd feel my boobies. I had imagined how I'd feel without them, but I didn't grasp the full weight of the situation yet. I tried to mentally and emotionally process what was to come, cupping them with my hands. I pictured them as conscious beings, having feelings about what was going to happen to them. Were they scared? Were they ready? I decided to write them a letter.

Dear Boobies,

You may not have fed babies or saved nations, but you have both served me well, and I thank you. You gave me a sense of femininity and power. I'm sorry that you're sick, that cancer is trying to eat you away. I'm sorry you've been overtaken by wonky cells. I never meant for this to happen. As we part tomorrow, we'll both go on to achieve a higher purpose. You'll go into a freezer at the university, part of research to help other women and other boobies. I'll go on living my life, boobless, and without cancer eating my body away. I don't know yet what my purpose in life is, but I'll do my best to find it. I promise. For you. For me. For us.

Love,
Emily

CHAPTER 35

FEELING THEM FOR THE LAST TIME

THE NEXT MORNING, July 16, I woke up later than usual, after Jonathan and Karen had already eaten breakfast. I didn't want to be around for that. I showered, got dressed, and gathered my fuzzy polar bear blanket and hospital bag. Dr. R anticipated that I'd stay one night before going home.

I chose to wear a mastectomy shirt to the hospital so it would be easy to put back on after surgery. It was a special shirt I bought online, made specifically for women healing from mastectomies. It buttoned up the front, so you didn't have to stretch out your arms to put it on. It also had internal pockets to hold drains, rubber bulbs that gathered the fluids produced by the body as it healed after surgery. Having these shirts was one of the tips I learned about from the social media groups.

Because of COVID-19 restrictions, I was allowed to bring only two people with me to the hospital. I chose to take Jonathan and Karen. Wayne planned to make himself busy by grocery shopping and running errands before swapping places with Karen at the hospital that evening.

"Are you ready?" Karen asked as we got into the car. I'm not sure if anyone is truly ready to have their boobs cut off.

"I think so," I said. "As ready as I'll ever be, I guess."

We arrived at the hospital, checked in, and sat in the waiting room. The nerves kicked in, so I laid my head on Jonathan's shoulder. Even though it was a hot summer day and I was already sweaty, his body heat against my face and his arm around my shoulder were comforting.

"Emily," a voice called through the waiting room. It was my turn.

"Here we go," I said as we got up and gathered our things.

We were led to a room with a hospital bed, presumably the one I'd be rolled away on. I put on the hospital gown, hair cap, and those socks with the rubber grips on the bottom. We waited in that room for what seemed like an hour. The hunger was setting in, and my patience was dwindling. A nurse finally came in to set up my IV.

"How much longer?" I asked in a sharp tone before catching myself. "I'm sorry. I don't mean to sound cranky. It's just that I'm hungry and nervous."

"It's normal to feel that way," she said. "And I'm not sure how long it'll be, but it shouldn't be too much longer. The surgeon is just closing another surgery, and she should be in here soon."

Just then, Dr. R and a group of other doctors walked in, including the anesthesiologist and the plastic surgeon. Even though I was having a flat closure, the plastic surgeon was going to perform a lymphovenous bypass. An article called "Lymphovenous Anastomosis Bypass Surgery" describes this procedure as a microsurgical technique where they attach residual lymphatic channels to a nearby vein. This allows the excess lymph fluid to reenter the body's circulation and reduces the risk of lymphedema after removing a person's lymph nodes. The plastic surgeon told me that I was the first she would be performing the surgery on prophylactically, as a preventive measure, as it was usually used as a treatment option after lymphedema had already occurred.

"How are you feeling?" Dr. R asked.

"I'm ready," I lied.

"I just want to double- and triple-check that you want both breasts removed," she said. "Once I take the healthy breast off, I can't put it back on, so I want to be extra sure before we go into the operating room."

"Yes," I said confidently. "I want both off." With so few options when it came to IBC treatment, this was the one choice I was able to make for myself. I wanted a double mastectomy for two reasons. First, I wanted additional peace of mind. I would never forgive myself if there was hidden cancer in my healthy boob, and I didn't do anything about it. I wanted all the breast tissue to be gone. The second reason was for symmetry. I wanted clothing to fit properly. I wanted to look and feel symmetrical.

"OK," Dr. R said as she finished marking up my boobs with a marker to indicate what to remove during surgery. "I'll let the other doctors talk with you, and we'll get you set up with anesthesia. I'll see you in there."

Dr. R left the room, and the anesthesiologist went over everything I should know. It wasn't my first time with anesthesia. I had several surgeries before and knew what to expect.

"Alright," she said. "It's time then. Let's get you back to the OR."

Jonathan reached down to give me a hug and a kiss, and the anesthesia team took over.

"You know," the anesthesiologist said as she rolled my bed down the hallway, "I think you're the calmest person we've had."

It was the same comment made by the team that put in my port. Except this time, I didn't feel calm. I was really nervous.

We got to the operating room, and I transferred to the operating table as music played and nurses bustled around preparing for the surgery. I saw the rubber breathing mask come out and knew the big moment was just a few seconds away.

"You ready?" the anesthesiologist asked.

"Hold on one second," I said, reaching down to feel my boobs. "I just wanted to feel them one last time." I crossed my arms and held my boobies for a few seconds.

"OK." I let go of them. "I'm ready."

She smiled at me sweetly, gave a nod, and placed the mask over my nose and mouth. I was out.

CHAPTER 36
I'M FLAT NOW

"I'M FLAT NOW. I'm flat *now*." The nurse rolled my bed down the hall to my hospital room, and I needed everyone around me to know I was flat now. Jonathan waited in the doorway to my room as he witnessed my sudden flat pride.

Still under the influence of some hard pain medication and the aftereffects of anesthesia, I gradually became aware of my surroundings in the room.

Jonathan sat on my right side, gently stroking my arm. I looked down and saw Karen and Wayne standing at the foot of the bed. *Wait a second*, I thought. *Wayne is here? I might be on drugs, but I know there are only supposed to be two visitors.*

"Whoa," I said in a breathy voice. "You're heeere."

"Yep," Jonathan said, rubbing my arm. "Everyone's here."

"But Wayne is here. *Whoa*." Wayne turned his face away to wipe tears from his eyes.

"Are you hungry?" a nurse asked. "Do you want something to eat?"

I was so surprised that the hospital had let three visitors into the room, I didn't notice she was standing next to me. "Yes," I replied. "I haven't eaten all day."

"Well, it's kind of late, so I'll see what I can find. Do you want a turkey sandwich?"

It was after eight, and the food services had already closed. I didn't care, though. Nothing sounded more delicious at that moment than a hospital turkey sandwich.

"Jonathan," I said as we waited for the food to arrive. "Take a picture."

"It's OK. We don't need a picture," he said.

"No," I snapped back. "Take a picture. I want documentation." I wanted a photo for proof, as if I would forget that my boobs had just been cut off. Not wanting to argue, Jonathan took out his phone to snap a selfie.

"What are you doing?" Karen said in a motherly tone. "Put that away. She's just waking up. It's not time for pictures."

"She wants documentation." He took a selfie of the two of us, me with my eyes glazed over and half open.

The nurse returned with a sandwich wrapped in plastic and a bowl of chicken noodle soup.

"Can Jonathan stay for the night?" I asked the nurse before she left the room. Overnight guests were still not allowed, but my medication-induced confidence asked anyway.

"I don't think that'll be a problem," she said. "Just keep it quiet because there aren't supposed to be overnight visitors." Jonathan wasn't expecting to stay overnight and wasn't prepared. He asked the nurse for a toothbrush. She also gave him a pillow and blanket to sleep on the couch under the window.

Karen and Wayne decided to head back to the house for the night. "We'll see you in the morning," Karen said. "Rest up."

After they left, I could barely keep my eyes open. I was so tired. But so hungry. Jonathan unwrapped the sandwich and started to feed me. I took a tiny bite and nibbled slowly as the sleepy weight of my eyes caused them to close. I felt myself slowly falling asleep with chewed-up bread and meat in my mouth.

"Fish," Jonathan said. "Wake up and swallow your food."

I opened my eyes and continued to chew. Over and over, I fell asleep while chewing, and Jonathan woke me up so I didn't choke. I don't know what happened to the soup.

CHAPTER 37
TWO OF EVERYTHING

"EMILY," A VOICE ECHOED in my head. "Wake up. It's time to get up and walk." I opened my eyes. The room was dark, and I could tell it was the middle of the night.

"What?" I asked, groggy and confused. I could barely make out two silhouettes backlit by the hallway's fluorescent lighting.

"It's time to get up and walk," the voice said again.

"What time is it?" I asked in a sleepy voice. "And where's Jonathan?" He was no longer beside the bed.

"It's about two o'clock," she said. "And your husband is asleep on the couch over there."

Satisfied that Jonathan was still in the room, I turned my attention back to the first thing she said. "Wait. You want me to get up and walk *now*? I don't think I can."

"You have to move around to start the healing process. And you have to try to use the bathroom. We're going to take out your catheter, OK?" I didn't know I had a catheter. They pulled back my blankets, and the nurse pulled out the catheter from my urethra.

"Owwww!" I yelled. I was definitely awake now.

They slowly turned my body as my legs draped over the side of the bed. Each nurse held an elbow as they lifted me to a standing position. All three of us slowly shuffled toward the bathroom.

Jonathan was still asleep. The female nurse stood beside me as I peed into a plastic container that sat inside the toilet bowl.

"Do I dump it?" I asked, not knowing what to do with the bucket of pee.

"No, I need to measure it first," she said. *Measure it? Weird, but OK*, I thought.

Getting back into bed was more difficult than getting out. I felt pressure across my chest and an ache in my armpit. My chest was wrapped up, and I suddenly became aware of the compression bra I was wearing and its zipper scratching my neck. Doing my best not to tear open any incisions, I methodically scooched my butt onto the bed and under my polar bear blanket and fell back asleep.

I woke up in the morning to sunlight pouring in through the hospital windows, more aware now that my chest and armpit had been sliced open the day before. The pain coming from my armpit drew my attention to my arm, and I noticed the compression sleeve on my arm and hand. *Was that there last night? I hadn't noticed.*

"Good morning, Fish," Jonathan said in a singsong voice as he smiled and rubbed my upper arm. He was sitting in the chair beside my bed again. "How do you feel?"

"Sore. Like someone ripped open my armpit."

"Well, they did," he joked. "Do you want coffee or food?"

"Oh my God, yes." I was desperate for a cup of coffee.

"I'll need to call to order. I'm hungry too, but I'm not supposed to be here, so I'll need to figure out how to get food."

"Just say it's for me," I said. "Pretend like I'm really hungry."

Jonathan picked up the phone to order breakfast. "Hi, good morning," he said. "Emily would like breakfast this morning. Yes, she'd like two coffees, two yogurts, two hash browns, and two orders of bacon."

I'm sure they believed him.

CHAPTER 38
FIRST LOOK

I WAS ALMOST FINISHED EATING when Karen and Wayne returned.

"How did you both get in here?" I asked now that I was fully awake.

"We just walked in like we belonged," Karen said. "If you act like you know what you're doing, nobody will question it."

As we were discussing how to skirt the rules, Dr. R walked in, along with her nurse and a medical resident. "Good morning," she said. "I came up to see how you're doing and to check your incisions."

"I feel pretty good. Just really sore in my armpit." My body was still loaded with narcotics, so the pain hadn't fully set in yet.

"That's expected," she said. "The plastic surgeon did a lot of work in there to reconnect your lymph vessels, so it'll be sore for a while. I'm happy to see you're wearing the compression sleeve. You'll need to wear that for six months since you had the lymphovenous bypass. It'll prevent lymphedema during the critical healing phase. I don't want you lifting your arm more than 90 degrees. Now let me take a look at your incisions."

The nurse helped her gently unwrap the dressings on my chest.

"Can I look?" I asked. "I want to see what it looks like."

"Are you sure you—"

Before she finished, I turned my head downward to see a flat chest with two straight incisions covered in surgical tape where my boobs used to be. "Wow. It looks so good. I'm so happy with it. It's just how I wanted it to look." I had been so scared of a botched mastectomy with lumps and bumps. But my chest was perfectly flat, and I felt a deep sense of relief.

"What's all this?" I asked, pointing at the clear tubes protruding from my sides. I had one tube coming out of my right side at the bra line, and two tubes coming out of the left side. Sitting on the bed next to me were three lemon-sized rubber balls holding a reddish-orange liquid. I realized that the fluid was my blood. I've never done well with the sight of my own blood, so I looked back up at the doctor.

"Those are your drains," Dr. R explained. "As you heal, you'll produce blood and fluid, and we don't want it to build up inside of you. Before you go, they'll teach you how to drain them and take care of them."

I had forgotten all about the drains. Seeing tubes coming out of my sides was disturbing. I was nervous about taking care of them.

"Don't worry," Karen chimed in from the corner of the room. "Jonathan and I will handle it."

The nurse wrapped my chest back up and put the compression bra back on. It was too big, though, and didn't do much compressing. It felt more like a loose vest.

Early that afternoon, after receiving my after-care instructions, Jonathan helped me sit up and put on the mastectomy shirt I arrived in as we waited for the wheelchair to arrive. I was going home. Without my boobs.

CHAPTER 39
CANCER-FREE

"DO YOU WANT TO GO OUT to celebrate?" Jonathan asked with a big grin on his face.

"Go out? Where?" I asked. "How am I supposed to go out?" I hadn't been out of the house since coming home from the hospital. I was still taking narcotics. Plastic tubes attached to drain bulbs still protruded from my sides.

"I was thinking we could just go to breakfast. It might feel good to get out of the house for a bit."

I agreed to go to breakfast but only because we were going to my favorite diner. Karen and Wayne came downstairs, ready to go. The drive to the restaurant was more comfortable than the ride home from the hospital had been.

Walking to our table, I felt like everyone's eyes were on me, like everyone knew I had tubes oozing blood and nasty fluid into rubber bulbs. I was self-conscious of my newly flat chest. The mastectomy shirt I was wearing wasn't exactly the epitome of high fashion. It was plain, medical, and homely. This wasn't how I imagined my boobless debut into society.

I was thankful to be seated toward the back of the restaurant, where few people could see us. I enjoyed my veggie scramble in peace until it was time to shuffle back to the front of the crowded diner.

Don't look at me. Don't look at me, I thought as I walked past the first few tables. Then something shifted inside of me. I could feel it emanating upward out of my soul. *You know what? Who cares? So I had surgery. Who cares if people see me in this horrid outfit? Who cares if people know I don't have boobs? Who cares? Not me. Not anymore.*

Later that afternoon, my phone rang.

"Hi, this is Dr. B. I have the pathology results from your mastectomy."

Jonathan and I went into the office for some privacy. I didn't want to be near anyone else if the results were bad. *Did they get all the cancer? Was there still cancer inside me? Would I need more surgery? Would I need more chemo?* My mind raced as I opened my notebook to write down everything the oncologist had to say.

"It looks like there were clear margins," she said. Good news so far. "The lymph nodes they took out were all clear, and the tumor is gone. But it looks like there was still a diffuse spread of cancer cells throughout the breast tissue."

I looked at Jonathan, wondering if he was as confused as I was. "What does that mean?" I asked.

"It's actually quite strange," Dr. B answered. "I've never seen this before, where the chemo takes care of the tumor but not the spread throughout the breast. So this means that the chemo didn't kill all the cancer."

"Oh," I said, feeling defeated as my heart sank and a sour taste filled my throat. "So what does that mean for me?" I expected her to give me a prognosis, to tell me I had six months to live if I was lucky. That all my suffering had been for nothing.

"It just means we have to shift things a little. Instead of having just immunotherapy, just Herceptin moving forward, you'll have immunotherapy mixed with chemo. It's called Kadcyla and was just approved by the FDA about two years ago. It's very promising. I think we talked about it when I first met you."

"So I need more chemo?" I was half asking and half processing this news to myself.

"Yes, but it's not like the other chemo. It's less intense. It'll still be every three weeks, but you won't feel like you did on TCHP. It's much better. And your hair will start to grow back. The tumor board has already met about your case, and we decided you'll need ten infusions. We want you to have a full year of treatment."

I did some quick math, counting out the weeks on my phone's calendar. Ten Kadcyla infusions would end nine days before the one-year anniversary of beginning chemotherapy.

"That's nine days less than a year," I said. "Can I do eleven so it's a full year?"

"Sure," she said. "Nobody's ever asked for more chemo, but that's fine with me if you feel better about it."

"I do," I replied. "And I have another question. I'm not sure if it's premature to ask this, though."

"Shoot," she said. "What's your question?"

"At what point might I be considered cancer-free? How will I know when all the cancer is gone?"

"I think it's safe to say that you're cancer-free right now." My eyes blinked through the tears welling up. I looked up at Jonathan. He wrote "cancer-free" in all capital letters on the notebook page.

"But I thought you said there was still cancer?" I asked.

"There was, but remember I told you there were clear margins," said Dr. B. "So the chemo didn't kill all of the cancer, but it was all removed at surgery. There is no known cancer in your body right now."

No known cancer.

"Oh my God," I said as the tears streamed down my face, racing toward my chin. "Thank you so much. Thank you, thank you, thank you."

It was officially one of the best days of my life.

CHAPTER 40

PEOPLE SAY WEIRD THINGS

PEOPLE CAN BE STRANGE. When friends and family found out I had cancer, some of them acted weird. Really weird. They said weird things. They did weird things. They sent me weird things.

Maybe we're never taught how to respond to tragic news. A lot of people don't know what to say when they hear that someone they know is sick or dying. In school, we're taught advanced math and the birthplace of Shakespeare as if we'll use that knowledge daily, but we're not taught empathy or compassion or people skills.

I don't fault most people for it. Some things are awkward. Sometimes people want to say the right thing but don't know what that is. And sometimes people don't think first and end up saying something strange, awkward, or even cruel. Following are some of my weirdest encounters.

"I hope you make it."

Me too, girl. Me too.

This might not seem bad, and it's not really. But when someone would say something like this, I always wondered, *As opposed to what?* This reminded me that I might *not* make it. I didn't like to think that I might not make it. I knew it, but I didn't want to be reminded of it.

"Everything happens for a reason."

No, it really doesn't. I understand that some people try to make meaning when something bad happens. But when it comes down to it, cancer is a group of wonky cells that quickly replicate. I always hated it when people would try to push their meaning-making agendas onto me. It isn't anyone else's job to tell me why something bad happened to me, or what life lesson I should take from it. That's for me to decide.

"Emilyyyyyyy! You're going to get lymphedema! Oh my Goddddd! Call me as soon as you get this."

Crying, wailing, and freaking out to someone who has just been diagnosed with cancer isn't supportive. It's terrifying. This was a message left on my voicemail.

The person who called to tell me this had gone through breast cancer more than twenty years prior. She had lymphedema as a result of outdated medical practices and not complying with doctors' orders after her mastectomy. When I listened to her message, my heart beat fast, and my hands began shaking. The fear in her voice was triggering, leading me straight into an anxiety attack.

Lymphedema is the swelling of an area, like an arm, after lymph nodes are removed from that region. In this case, if there is cancer in the lymph nodes surrounding the breast, those nodes are removed. Because they're gone, lymphatic fluid has nowhere to be processed and can build up in the arm, causing swelling and pain. It's not fun.

Science has also changed in the twenty years since she had surgery. There are now techniques and procedures to avoid extreme lymphedema, like the lymphovenous bypass surgery I had along with the double mastectomy.

Even though I had this procedure, there was a chance I could still get lymphedema. And there was a chance I wouldn't. There was no way to know. What I did know was that I would comply with every little instruction the doctors, surgeons, and physical therapists gave me. And I won't call anyone to scream and cry to them and tell them they're going to get lymphedema.

I did not call her back.

"I don't mean to sound insensitive, but at least you don't have kids."

Both parts of this statement grind my gears because both are weird and insensitive.

When someone says that they don't mean to sound insensitive, judgmental, mean, or whatever, they sound *more* insensitive by acknowledging that they know it sounds insensitive. By saying it anyway, it sounds like they don't give a flying rat's ass about compassion.

I didn't have kids. Sure, I was thirty-five years old. My eggs were probably deteriorating. I wanted kids, even though life's circumstances didn't agree. Jonathan and I had wanted to try for a biological child in our twenties. It was perfect timing, or so we thought. Then it didn't happen. So we decided we would adopt. We had both felt drawn to adoption, even before we met. We both always thought we'd adopt a child. The point is, you don't know anyone's past with fertility or if they do or don't want children. And all choices are valid.

I fully acknowledge that having young children while undergoing treatment adds a layer of complication. They are small humans who rely on you. Someone needs to take care of them. It's impossible to take care of yourself during cancer treatment, let alone the twenty-four-seven needs of a developing person. I sympathize with how difficult that must be.

The unsaid, implied meaning of saying something like "at least you don't have children" suggests that at least if I died, I wouldn't be leaving a child motherless. I'm sure someone could write a completely different book about how messed up it is that a woman's life is somehow less valuable if she is not a mother. Childless women are people and have people who love them and care about them, adults and children alike.

As Tracee Ellis Ross once said, "The childless women have been mothering the world and elevating culture as aunties, godmothers, teachers, mentors, sisters, and friends, and the list goes on. And you do not need to push out a baby to help push humanity forward."

There are children in my life whom I love just as much as if they were my own—nieces, nephews, friends' children.

Everyone has people who love and care about them. And if you think you don't have someone who cares about you, you do. Because I love and care about you.

"My grandma / aunt / friend's cousin's third-grade teacher had that. And she died."

If I had a dollar for every person who said this to me, I could buy at least a decent cup of coffee. Several friends and family members had the mind to tell me about everyone they knew who died from the same disease I was just diagnosed with.

First, I'm sorry for your loss.

Second, letting me know of people who passed away from the same type of cancer that is devastating my body is not helpful. It only reminds me that I might die of this, too. I already know this. I don't need to be reminded of it. But thank you for trying to relate.

"Have you tried doing essential oils about it?"

Look, I'm all about alternative medicine. I believe everything has its place. And I love essential oils. They smell amazing. As a self-identified woo-woo girl, I love collecting crystals, oils, and analyzing astrology and numerology for fun. But let's be clear. When it comes to life-threatening diseases, the only correct answer is science. Researched, peer-reviewed, proven science. As far as I'm aware, nobody has beaten IBC using alternative medicine alone. However, I know several women who chose that path and have sadly passed away. So while alternative therapies can complement modern medicine, it is important to understand the aggressiveness and urgency of IBC.

Reiki for oncology is often used for symptom management. This is an appropriate use of alternative healing as a complement to conventional medicine. Similar to acupuncture and massage therapy, these modalities can help to temporarily relieve symptoms but will not cure cancer. Neither will essential oils.

"Hey, at least you'll get new boobs."

Are you sitting down? I have some bad news. I'm not getting new boobs.

Any statement that begins with "at least" lacks empathy. It diminishes the other person's experience and invalidates what they may be feeling. There are no "at leasts" with cancer or any other challenge in life.

Not only does this imply that boobs are necessary appendages, it assumes that I'll be eligible to receive reconstruction of some sort. It also suggests that "new" boobs are equal to or better than natural breasts.

I don't fault people for not knowing their post-mastectomy options. I didn't know of the reconstruction possibilities until I was faced with breast cancer. However, not all options are good options or even possible options. There are breast implants of multiple varieties, DIEP flap procedures (where they take fat and tissue from other parts of your body and re-create a breast shape with it), flat aesthetic closure, and more of which I'm likely unaware.

Those with inflammatory breast cancer are not eligible for reconstruction until several years after surgery. Because the cancer affects the skin, the surgeon must remove as much of it as possible, leaving no extra skin for an implant or relocated body fat to occupy.

In hindsight, I'm glad I wasn't eligible for reconstruction right away because I would have chosen it. Being flat has introduced me to other women who have received flat aesthetic closures. Some are like me, not eligible for reconstruction. Others had reconstruction and later chose to go flat for various reasons. These are some of the most beautiful people I know, and I'm grateful to be in the flattie community with them.

"You should get nipples tattooed on."

Didn't your parents tell you that you shouldn't tell other people what to do? And why do you care so much about my nipples? That's weird.

Do I need nipples to be more of a woman or more of a person? No. Mind your business.

"I'm feeling stronger every day."

This statement was said by an internet friend who was going through the same type of chemotherapy that I was. The breast cancer community can feel small at times, especially among those who are going through treatment simultaneously. We rely on each other for support and to feel less alone. At the end of the day, nobody can truly know what this kind of treatment feels like unless they've experienced it themselves.

This friend also received TCHP and often said that she was feeling stronger every day. In addition to saying this to me, she shared this sentiment on social media. I wanted to scream, "Girl, you are *not* feeling stronger every day!"

Chemotherapy doesn't work like that. Chemotherapy is poison. It destroys fast-reproducing cells, and it does not discriminate between cancer cells and your body's healthy cells. This is why chemo patients feel so ill and experience terrible side effects. It makes you feel weaker and sicker every day. Given enough chemotherapy, a person will die.

Most chemotherapy is also cumulative, meaning it builds up in your system over time. A person feels worse the farther along in treatment they are. It doesn't get better. It gets worse. That's science.

I don't know why my friend would say that it made her feel stronger. Maybe to make her friends and family feel better? Maybe she didn't want them to know she was suffering?

There are so many dangers to telling a lie like this. Others reading it are going through the same thing, like I was. If she befriended me, I assume she befriended others, too, and they were reading it as well. I also presume, based on statistics, that she has friends and family who will also go through a breast cancer diagnosis one day.

Saying things like that can make others feel like they're doing something wrong when they feel like complete shit on chemo. When I read those words, I thought, *Why does she feel stronger, and I feel like my organs are shutting down? Why does she feel good, and I feel like shit?* Then I realized she was lying. It wasn't true.

Saying you're feeling good when you're really not is not only a lie, it's irresponsible. And it's cruel. Don't do it.

Funeral Cards

Shortly after I lost my hair, I received a message from a distant relative. I hadn't met this person before. I didn't know her, and she didn't know me. In her message, she told me she was sending me something in the mail. I thought that was sweet of her. Until it came.

I opened the package and took out the note.

I saw this photo on your Facebook page, and I thought you looked strong. I had these cards printed and thought you could hand them out. I've already given them to members of our family.

Excuse me? You did what now? She and I weren't connected on social media, so she had to purposefully look me up and snag a public photo.

The cards were printed with my face from a picture I once used on my profile. I was doing a challenge, wearing a dress every day to raise awareness and money to support survivors of human trafficking. I had taken a photo to show off one of the outfits. Wearing a dress every day isn't as simple as it seems, especially when you don't own a lot of dresses, but still want a fresh look every day. Accessorizing and styling are essential, and I was proud of the outfit I had put together. I was also proud of the amount of money I raised to support survivors. She had pilfered the photo and had it printed on cards.

What was I supposed to do with this? I imagined walking up to someone and saying, *Here, guys. Take this card. It's a picture of me when I was healthy and had hair. Remember me the way this distant cousin thinks I should be remembered, OK?*

It reminded me too much of a funeral card, except without the prayer, and felt incredibly disturbing. It especially upset my mother.

I'm still not sure what the point of that was. It was weird. I eventually met her briefly a couple of years later at a family event. There was no mention of the funeral cards.

> "It's always something. You're using your cancer as an excuse (to not think about me)."

Sometimes the people closest to you are the cruelest. This truth is something I was unprepared for. This statement was said shortly after I became cancer-free. Let's call this person Sadie for the sake of this story. That's not her real name, of course.

Sadie was going through a rough patch in her personal life, and I felt compassion for her. During the same time, I had a massive cancer scare and was receiving scans to determine if the cancer had spread to my bones. I had severe rib pain with no explanation and was terrified. If it had spread, I'd be reclassified as stage IV and terminal.

I hadn't mentioned the pain or scans to anyone other than Jonathan and my mom. I didn't want anyone to worry unnecessarily until I knew for sure what was happening. So I stayed to myself. I didn't socialize. I didn't talk to friends much. I just stayed in my house with my cats and kept to myself. Maybe that was my fault, especially since I had been so publicly open previously.

Then one day, I learned that Sadie had removed me from her social media. She removed Jonathan, too. Me being me, I wasn't going to let it go. If I unknowingly did something to offend her, I wanted to apologize and make it right. Both Jonathan and I had been close to Sadie. It was very strange that we'd just be cut out of her life.

I texted Sadie to ask why she removed us from social media and to ask if she was OK. To paraphrase, she was upset that I hadn't reached out to her during the hard time she was going through. I apologized up and down, explaining that I had been going through a cancer scare, was caught up in my own fears and issues, but was very sorry for not reaching out.

"It's too late for apologies," she said. "It's always something. You're using cancer as an excuse when you should have reached out to me to ask how I'm doing."

In that moment, I felt like she was dismissing my life. My living, breathing self. I felt like she was saying she didn't care if I lived or died. Her issue was more important. I was devastated.

Looking back at text messages from the previous year, I realized that she never asked how I was doing during my diagnosis or chemotherapy. She didn't inquire about my well-being while I was at my sickest. The only communication from her was to complain about the other people in my life. I then realized this relationship wasn't what I thought, and I moved on, focusing on people who are interested in a two-way relationship. At the time of writing this, Sadie and I are no longer close and rarely communicate.

The scan ended up being clear. The cancer hadn't spread. Sadie didn't care.

Nothing

There were a few family members and lifelong friends who said nothing at all. This was painful. Sometimes saying nothing is more hurtful than saying something weird or awkward or cruel. Maybe they didn't know what to say, so they said nothing at all. I choose to believe this is the case.

CHAPTER 41
PEOPLE SAY SUPPORTIVE THINGS

WHILE SOME PEOPLE respond to a cancer diagnosis unthoughtfully or strangely, others are incredibly loving and supportive. May we all learn how to lovingly respond to someone with cancer or other life-changing challenges.

"I don't know what to say, but I want you to know that I care, and I'm thinking of you."

This may be the most thoughtful thing a friend said to me after my diagnosis. Admitting that you don't know what to say is vulnerable. Sometimes there isn't a perfect thing to say, but acknowledging that you care is most important.

"This really sucks."

The empathy in this statement is spot-on. It does suck. It's awful. Sitting in the suck with someone is one of the most caring and empathetic things you can do.

"I know we haven't talked in a really long time, and I hope this isn't weird. But I want you to know I'm thinking of you."

Not weird at all! Sometimes it's the hard things that bring people back together. Reconnecting with old friends was one of the best things that came from having cancer. Not only did I discern what was important in life and what wasn't, but others did as well. In the end, love is the most important thing.

"Do you want to video chat? I'd love to hang out with you."

Because of my compromised immune system, seeing people in person wasn't a great idea. COVID-19 and other viruses were running rampant in the community. A video chat was the perfect solution to spend time together while keeping germs away. It's also great for long-distance loved ones to show they care. I could never promise I'd be very jovial or fresh-looking, but sometimes it was good to see a friend and talk about normal, non-cancer things. I appreciated the company and the distraction.

"What's your address? I want to send you something."

Look, as long as it isn't my own funeral card, send me whatever you want. Physical gifts aren't very important to me. Words of affirmation and quality time are more my love language. But I know that gifts are how a lot of people show they care. And I can appreciate that. After all, a person can never have too many blankets.

"I'm praying for you / sending you good vibes."

I'm all about that positive energy! Any positive energy that was sent my way, whether through prayer, vibes, meditation, Reiki, or anything else, was so appreciated. Giving someone your time and energy through positive intention is a precious gift.

Phyllis

My grandmother Phyllis wasn't my grandmother. She was my great-great-aunt through marriage.

Phyllis unofficially adopted my mother and me when my biological grandparents weren't around. Phyllis was the most consistent older woman in my life since the beginning. And because the other kids around me called her Grandmom, she was my Grandmom, too. She was my grandmother in every sense except DNA.

Phyllis was a firecracker. She was a military wife who raised five children. Her husband served in World War II, Vietnam, and Korea. She survived tuberculosis back when people didn't survive tuberculosis. She was an avid animal lover who had dogs, cats, birds, and even a squirrel. She would always tell me, *Never turn away anyone in need, people or pets.* And she didn't.

Phyllis was also a breast cancer survivor. Hers was caught in its early stages by a mammogram screening, and she didn't need the harsh treatments that I did. But she knew the feelings that came with a diagnosis.

If anyone in this world understood the challenges I faced as a military wife and now a cancer survivor, it was her. We grew close over the years as she would tell stories about her own military wife days, often twelve or thirteen times, because she'd forget that she had already told them. She had stories for days, as most people with her level of life experience do.

The last time I saw her was in early 2020, just before the world shut down due to the pandemic, and traveling was ill-advised. When I was diagnosed with cancer, Grandmom was going through her own battle with kidney disease. She rarely spoke of it because she didn't want me to worry. But I knew she was struggling. However, that didn't stop her from stepping up to the plate to support me.

She called me and wrote letters almost every week.

Her final letter was on stationery printed with an image of a kitten in a field of chamomile flowers. Even now, I look back at it in awe that she had the heart to support me through her own failing health.

> *Hi Emily – I know you're going through a lot right now, and I feel so bad 'cause there's nothing I can do to help except my prayers. You know they're always with you! It's not like when you were a little girl and had a boo-boo. A kiss could make it all better (& maybe a [B]and-aid). If it would help, I'd send a carton full! All I can say is just stay strong. We're all pulling for you and love you so much. Bye for now!*
>
> *Love,*
> *Grandmom*

Phyllis passed away at the age of ninety-two, soon after I completed cancer treatment. She left knowing her prayers were answered.

CHAPTER 42
SNAKE UNDER MY SKIN

RECEIVING NEWS that I was cancer-free, but still needed more chemo, was very strange. On the surface, it made no sense. Why would someone who doesn't have cancer anymore need more chemo? The reasoning was that if there was still cancer in the tissue that was removed, there might still be rogue cancer cells lurking around my body. HER2-positive cancers are aggressive, and recent studies published in *The New England Journal of Medicine* showed that stage III patients who received Kadcyla following a partial response to chemotherapy, as opposed to immunotherapy alone, were 50 percent less likely to experience breast cancer recurrence or death due to breast cancer.

While making sense of being cancer-free yet still needing chemo was on my mind until my next infusion, I had other things to handle first.

Ten days after surgery, I had my follow-up appointment with Dr. R to check on the healing process. I showed her the piece of paper on which I had tracked the amount of fluid being output into the drains. Karen and Jonathan squeezed my drain tubes and emptied the bulbs twice a day. I was responsible for writing down how much blood and fluid had collected, along with their color. It was gross. Dr. R took the paper and looked it over. Then she checked how my incisions were healing. The surgical tape holding me together was peeling along the outside edges.

"Your incisions look really good," she said. "You're healing really well. I think that tape will fall off completely in the next few days. We can get those drains out today."

This was music to my ears. The drains had become painful, irritating my skin where they were sewn into my body. I took a narcotic pain pill that morning in preparation for the drains being removed. I didn't know what to expect but was worried it might be painful.

Dr. R wished me happy healing and left the room. Meredith, her nurse, prepared the space with scissors and other sterile equipment. She snipped the stitches that held the drains in and prepared me for what was to come.

"OK, take a deep breath," she instructed. "And when you breathe out, I'm going to pull." Jonathan sat in the chair directly across from me, leaning forward and watching intently. "Big breath in. And out." I exhaled as she pulled. I kept my sight on Jonathan's face for composure.

The tube ran under my skin, through my chest, and around in a circle where my boob used to be. Jonathan looked as if he was watching an alien abduction in real time, his wide eyes fixed on my chest.

"Are you OK?" I asked him.

"Are *you* OK?" he asked back. "That looked like a snake moving under your skin."

"How was it?" Meredith asked. "Did it hurt, or are you OK?"

"I'm OK. It felt weird but didn't hurt. I'm glad I took that pain pill."

She repeated the process for the next two drains. Breathe in, breathe out, snake under the skin.

When the last drain came out, and tubes were no longer tethered to me, I felt like a brand-new woman.

CHAPTER 43
THE IN-LAWS ARE LEAVING

THAT NIGHT, Wayne took dinner requests. With my drains out and healing in full effect, there wasn't much for them to help with anymore. They would be leaving the next day.

Jonathan and I both requested turkey cutlets with salad, our favorite meal during their visit. Wayne had cooked every meal during their stay, and I was grateful. I know Jonathan appreciated the break as well. I was also thankful to finally taste food again, as it was meant to taste. Not metallic, or bland, or indescribably different. It had been more than a month since systemic chemotherapy had destroyed my taste buds, and their function was finally returning.

As Karen and Wayne hauled their luggage down the stairs and gathered it by the door the next morning, a feeling of sadness washed over me. We'd had company almost constantly for the last five months. I didn't know if we were ready to be on our own, but we were about to find out.

Jonathan and I returned home from the airport, took a breath, and looked at each other. It was just us. There were no visitors or helpers planned for the rest of the treatment process. We were on our own again. Although I was less than confident about being able to take care of myself, I looked forward to trying.

I made it my job to rest. My body needed to heal from the trauma of surgery and its aftermath. The surgical tape continued to peel back every day, revealing more of the incisions. The edges of my skin aligned, and it looked like someone had drawn two perfect lines across my chest.

As the pain lessened, I was able to climb in and out of bed without Jonathan's help. Showering by myself for the first time in months felt incredible. I had a newfound sense of freedom, even if it was just taking care of my basic needs. My mind began to remember what being independent felt like.

I desired to be independent and capable again. I hated relying on people to do basic tasks like bathing, dressing myself, cooking, and preparing my medication. I hated that my brain didn't work like it used to. I couldn't retain information after reading a simple paragraph. I didn't trust myself to pay bills, worried that I might mess something up or forget what I was doing mid-task and not complete it.

But now those things were coming back to me. I could dress myself again without help. I could stand long enough in front of the stove to cook a meal. If I took my time, I could retain information while reading. This would take more time and patience, but progress was happening. Even with little improvements, I felt a sense of accomplishment. I felt hope, like regaining complete independence was possible if I took it one step at a time, one day at a time. Maybe one day I'd be able to do all the things I could do before cancer. That was the dream.

Just as I was feeling a new sense of "normal," it was time to undergo more treatment. I wondered if it would ever end. Where was the light at the end of the tunnel?

CHAPTER 44
MORE CHEMO

MY FIRST KADCYLA infusion was scheduled for Jonathan's birthday. That wasn't on purpose, but his birthday fell on the next Tuesday during the three-week infusion interval.

"I'm so sorry. Do you want me to see if I can change it?" I asked him. I felt awful that he'd have to be at the clinic on his special day.

"No, it's fine," he said. "It might be nice to have off work that day."

While most of the TCHP infusions were in Salt Lake City, where Dr. B held her appointments, my Kadcyla treatments would be at the infusion center closest to our house. These infusions didn't require a doctor's visit beforehand, and the convenience of a shorter drive was a nice change of pace. It was at the same clinic where I received my first TCHP infusion, and I was hoping to see Jackie again.

I arrived with my blanket, my big pink water bottle, and a bag of snacks. As Jonathan and I settled in, a nurse entered our curtained-off pod. It wasn't Jackie.

"Hi, I'm Heather. I'm going to be your infusion nurse today. Can I get you anything while we wait for the pharmacy to make your medication?"

"No, thank you." I tried not to sound disappointed. "I think we're good for now. Is Jackie working today? I was hoping to say hi."

"I'm sorry, Jackie doesn't work here anymore," she replied. "I'm actually her replacement."

This news hit deep within my heart. I felt like crying. Jackie was the first fellow-TCHP patient I had met, and her current state of being—her beauty and vibrant energy—had given me hope. I wanted to thank her for that. "That's OK," I said with a forced smile.

Heather unwrapped the sterile pack of equipment and accessed my port, leaving the tube hanging from my chest while I waited. Jonathan set up his work laptop, and I opened a game of Candy Crush on my phone. All of this had become routine by now.

A short time later, Heather opened the curtain. "It's here. Are you ready for your first Kadcyla?"

"I don't need pre-meds first?" I asked. Nobody had given me steroids or anti-nausea medication yet. I always had steroids and anti-nausea medication before chemo.

"Not for this," she said. "This one is much less intense than the chemo you had before. I think you'll find that you can tolerate it much better."

"I hope you're right." I was hesitant as she turned to the nurse who was attempting my long, complicated last name while verifying my identity. Heather put on the yellow hazmat equipment and attached the bag of chemo to the IV pole and into my port. I reclined the chair, put in my earbuds, and jammed out to Taylor Swift for an hour.

The familiar beeping of the IV pump let me know that the hour was up. *Wow. That was fast.* I had gotten used to spending the entire day at the clinic. An hour felt like a walk in the park.

"You did it," Heather said as she entered the room. "I just need to flush your port, and you're good to go." We were home by lunchtime.

The next few days felt nothing like the first week after TCHP. I was exhausted and had throat nausea, a tickling sensation at the back of my throat that made me want to gag, but I didn't feel like I was dying.

I can totally do this, I thought.

CHAPTER 45
RADIATION

JUST AS THE PEACH FUZZ began emerging from my scalp, I prepared for the next big phase of treatment: radiation. Radiation and Kadcyla would run concurrently, and I worried about days when I'd have both on the same day. How would that make me feel? Would I be completely wiped out? That was a bridge to cross when we got there.

Before meeting with the radiation team, a friend thought it might be helpful to talk with her other friend, who was a breast cancer survivor. She assured me her friend was amazing and wanted to help, so I accepted the offer. I was taken aback, though, when this woman sent me a message that said "Please do your research. I know someone who chose radiation, and she now has coronary heart disease." I audibly gasped after reading her words. I didn't know anyone who had gone through radiation, and this was the first advice I got. *Don't do it or your heart will be diseased.* I was terrified.

After some social media stalking, I learned that she had been diagnosed with a very early stage of breast cancer and didn't need all the complex treatment that an IBC patient requires. I wanted to shout *You don't know me!* through my phone. Hearing that I could become gravely ill while trying to achieve a cure felt completely derailing and demoralizing. I was trying to be positive, to have hope, to be optimistic. I didn't want to consider every way these lifesaving treatments could go wrong.

As someone with IBC, I had no choice. Radiation was part of the standard IBC protocol, and I *had* to do it. Research performed by the Institut Curie showed that the five-year recurrence-free survival rate for non-metastatic IBC patients who received radiation was more than 85 percent. This was a significant part of the protocol. So it's what I would do.

I met with Dr. K, my radiation oncologist, the day after my first Kadcyla infusion. She was a tall, thin woman with a straight-to-the-point bedside manner. There was no head stroking or hand-holding like there was with Dr. B. She was kind, but direct. She explained the radiation process and that I would need to have treatment every weekday for thirty days, only resting on the weekends. Then she asked if I had any questions.

"Yes," I responded. "Does radiation cause heart disease?"

"It's possible, but not common," she said. "Especially with women who have breast cancer on the left side because it's close to your heart. But we have techniques now to prevent that from happening. Are you still having regular echocardiograms?"

"Yes," I said. I had an echocardiogram every three months to make sure chemo didn't damage my heart.

"Great. Those can detect early signs of any heart issues. We'll also see if you're a candidate for breath holds."

"Breath holds?" I asked. "What's that?"

"It's called a Deep Inspiration Breath Hold," Dr. K said. "It helps protect the heart from radiation, and they'll be able to see if you're a candidate during your planning session. That's when we'll fit you for your body mold. It'll keep you still so you don't move during treatments. They'll give you your radiation schedule at that time, too."

Deep Inspiration Breath Hold (DIBH) is a technique used while breast cancer patients receive radiation treatment. Holding a deep breath while receiving radiation therapy is one of many techniques used to help physicians reduce the amount of radiation that reaches the heart.

"Do you know when the planning session will be?" I asked.

"In about two weeks." Dr. K looked down at her notes. "We'll have to check the schedule."

"Oh," I said. I had already looked at the calendar and was hoping for an earlier start date. "You see, my brother's wedding is in Pennsylvania at the end of October, and Jonathan is the best man. I think I'll be cutting it close if I'm supposed to have six weeks of treatment. I want to make sure I'm finished with radiation before then. I really want to go to my brother's wedding."

"Hmm," she said, beginning to write something down. "Let me see if we can get you in sooner then. That's an important life event. We wouldn't want you to miss it."

My body relaxed with relief. All I wanted to do was be there for my brother's big day.

One week later, I took my first steps into the radiation department at Huntsman Cancer Institute in Salt Lake City. It was planning day.

A friendly radiation technician with perfectly coiffed blond hair had me change into a hospital gown and guided me into the room where my body would be mapped for treatments. A CT machine filled most of the cramped space. To the side was a smaller room with a viewing window that looked into the room where I was. People were everywhere, bustling about like a complicated but well-orchestrated symphony.

I sat on the CT machine table, and a curly-haired technician greeted me. She was working closely with Mr. Coif.

"We're going to fit you for your mold first," she explained. "Then we're going to see if you're a candidate for breath holds." She picked up a purple-ink pen and started marking the left side of my chest. "I'm just making some marks to indicate the radiation field."

When she finished, it was time to take the impression for the body mold. Because the radiation field would include my armpit, I lifted my left arm above my head as I lay back. I then sank into a warm, squishy plastic bag full of a gel-like substance. It felt like a huge heat pack used for period cramps, except it was the size of my entire upper body. I did my best to stay perfectly still while the mold set. This was the position I'd be in during every radiation session, and we needed to make sure it was right. I didn't want to mess everything up by moving.

"We're going to test out those breath holds now," Mr. Coif said. "How are you at holding your breath for a long time?"

I had spent my childhood in Grandmom's backyard, throwing rubber rings into the deep end of the swimming pool and holding my breath while I dived down to retrieve them. I also played the clarinet through elementary and middle school. I liked to think I had a good set of lungs on me.

"Pretty good," I said confidently.

"That's good. Because we're going to need you to hold your breath for as long as you can. I'll be talking to you through the speaker, letting you know when you can breathe."

Mr. Coif joined the rest of the staff behind the glass window as I lay on the CT machine's cold metal table.

"OK, when you're ready," he said through the speaker, "take a deep breath and hold it for as long as you can." I filled my lungs with as much air as I could and held it. And held it. And held it.

"Breathe," he said. "That was really good. I'll be right in there." He returned with Ms. Curly Hair. "The doctor is going to look at those images and see if your heart moved out of the way."

"Do you have any tattoos?" Ms. Curly Hair asked as we waited for the doctor.

"No," I answered. "No tattoos." I assumed she was asking because maybe having tattoos affected radiation somehow, but that wasn't why.

"So I'll be giving you your first tattoos?" she said with a wide grin. "How exciting!"

"What?" I was confused. "Why am I getting tattoos?"

"It's so we align the machine to your body the same exact way every time," she said. "The radiation field is very precise. We don't want to accidentally radiate your thyroid or heart, so we want it to be exact. We use little tattooed dots to do that."

Until then, I hadn't given any thought to my thyroid or if it might be irradiated into oblivion. I was glad someone else was thinking about that. As she prepared my skin, the doctor entered the room with a smile.

"Good news. You're an excellent candidate for breath holds. The only annoying part is you'll have to come to the main hospital for every session."

"Every single day?" I raised my eyebrows, hoping I had heard him wrong. The main hospital of Huntsman was near downtown Salt Lake City on the bench of the Wasatch Mountains. It was a forty-five-minute drive from my house. This was much farther than the satellite clinics where I had received my chemotherapy treatments.

"Yes," he confirmed. "We only have one machine that works with breath holds, and that's where it is."

"Ready for your first tattoo?" Ms. Curly Hair interrupted. First tattoos don't stop for inconvenient news.

"Go for it," I said. I didn't feel a thing as she poked four pin-sized tattoos over the markings she made earlier.

On my way out, one of the nurses from behind the window handed me a piece of paper with my radiation schedule. I would need to be at the hospital every morning by eight. Good thing I was a morning person.

CHAPTER 46
BURNT TO A CRISP

THE MORNING OF my first radiation session, I was so nervous that I gave myself double the necessary time to get to the hospital. Like on the first day of a new job, I was paranoid about being late. I was so early that I waited in the parking garage for almost an hour until my appointment time. It turns out there's not much traffic while most of the city is still asleep.

I checked in, and a nurse showed me to the women's changing room and then to the women's waiting room. Women and men had separate waiting rooms. Both had huge windows looking into the hallway, so I'm not sure why the waiting rooms were kept separate. They weren't private. We could see each other.

My name was called, and a radiation technician named Jennifer led me down the hall. Jennifer was the head radiation technician on my team. She didn't introduce herself that way, but I could tell by her interaction with the other techs. She was in charge. She stopped at a desk outside the room where I'd receive radiation.

"Every day, we'll stop here, and you'll tell us your full name and birthday," she told me. "We check to make sure we're giving the proper treatment to the right person. Then we'll head this way."

Jennifer led me through a set of double doors, down a long hallway, and into a large cold room with a huge machine

I had never seen before. It had a giant rotating arm attached to a sterile-looking metal table. I assumed that's where I'd be lying. Another tech pulled my body mold out of a storage cabinet.

"Today might take a little longer than usual because we're getting everything set up," Jennifer explained. "But it should only take about ten minutes every day."

I sat on the cold table and dropped the hospital gown to my waist. I lay down and raised my left arm over my head, tilting my head to the right. My body found its place in the contours of the mold. *Like a glove*, I thought.

Three techs surrounded me as they adjusted my torso, aligning the tattoos with the laser-like beams shining from the machine. They put a shiny fabric, called a bolus, on the left side of my chest where the cancer had been. The bolus material increased the dose sent to the skin, an area of great concern for those with IBC.

Then everyone left the room. I was suddenly alone in this sterile-feeling room with dimmed lights and laser beams illuminating my chest. It felt like some kind of torture scene from a sci-fi movie. Jennifer's voice came over the intercom.

"OK, when you're ready, take a deep breath and hold it." With my head tilted, I could see a computer monitor light up. There was a graph on the screen that moved every time I took a breath. I wondered if they were looking at the same screen on their end to make sure my breath hold was good enough. As I inhaled, the graph swelled and turned red.

"Let out just a little bit of air," Jennifer's voice said. I exhaled slightly, and the graph became green. *Aha*, I thought. *The graph is the guide.* I tried hard to stay perfectly still, not moving any organs inside my body. "OK, you can breathe."

Another technician came into the room and adjusted the settings on the machine. She left just as fast as she came in. I paid attention to the graph on the screen again as I repeated the breath hold. Jennifer walked into the room.

"That's it," she said. "You did a great job. You're done for today and can head back to the changing room. We'll see you tomorrow."

I saw them the next day. And the day after. And the day after.

In addition to the staff, I saw the same patients in the waiting room each morning. As *Golden Girls* played on the TV in the corner of the room, another screen showed the status of each radiation room and if it was delayed for any reason. Sometimes the fellow patients made small talk.

Is anyone waiting for a delayed room? The most I ever waited was thirty minutes.

How is the weather today? It was early fall, and the weather was usually great.

Does anyone have any vacations coming up? I loved hearing about the vacations people were planning since I wasn't allowed to travel yet.

How's everyone holding up with their treatment? After all, we all had cancer.

Susan finishes treatment today. I was always happy for anyone who announced it was their last day. Go you!

One early morning, it was just one other woman and me in the waiting room. She had long curly dark hair, and it was obvious she hadn't gone through chemo before her radiation treatments.

"How are you holding up?" she asked.

"I mean, it hurts. I'm pretty burnt. How are you doing?"

"Oh man, I'm struggling," she replied. "My bra is rubbing against the redness of where the radiation is. I don't know how I'm going to do the next three sessions."

"How many sessions do you need?" I asked, wondering how she was only experiencing redness with just three sessions to go.

"Seven. How about you?"

"Thirty," I said. "You're lucky to have redness. My skin is falling off. I have second-degree burns."

She stared at me, unblinking in astonishment. I didn't want to minimize her experience, but it was then that I realized not all cancer patients understand what it's like to go through the full spectrum of treatment. Sometimes I feel mean saying this because all cancer is bad and scary. No cancer is good. But we're not all the same. We don't all have the same experience, even in cancer treatment. Some people have a lumpectomy, a relatively minor breast surgery, and a few doses of radiation that turn their skin red. And some people are filled with poison, have their body parts amputated, and are burned to a literal crisp. Every woman in that room may have had cancer, but our experiences were not equal. I found myself feeling jealous of those who didn't know what this was like.

With burns on the left side of my chest and in my armpit, my body tissue was weeping. Every day, I covered my oozing chest in prescription burn cream. I used layers of gauze and soft fabric, along with a six-inch-wide Ace bandage wrapped around my torso like a mummy. I didn't want my body leaking all over my clothes. It hurt like hell, and I counted down the days until it was over.

As my chest became more and more burned by the day, it became increasingly difficult to raise my left arm above my head during the sessions. The skin was stiff, and I worried it would crack open even more if I pushed it too far. To distract me as she helped me force it slowly into place, Jennifer asked if I had ever gone to the Disney parks.

"Oh my gosh. I love Disney." I told her about the YouTube videos I watched during chemo, daydreaming about the day I'd visit again.

"I'm going to Disney World with my family next week," she told me.

"That's awesome," I said. "I'm planning a trip to Disneyland when I'm finished with treatment. Like a celebration thing."

"You should totally do it. What's your favorite ride?"

"Soarin'," I replied. I loved the free feeling of flying over beautiful scenery and landmarks around the world. The thought was especially appealing at this moment.

Before I knew it, my arm was in place, and it was time to hold my breath and be radiated again. We continued this routine every day, and every day, I dreaded the next. The pain was excruciating, but it wasn't going to last forever. There were only a few days left.

I was happy I was assigned early morning appointments. Not only was the traffic good, but it also allowed me to take afternoon naps. Radiation is exhausting, and I was still receiving Kadcyla every three weeks. I was extremely fatigued. Until then, I was never much of a nap person. I hated naps. They messed up my circadian rhythm, and I didn't like that. I valued my sleep schedule. Radiation zapped the energy out of me, though. I napped almost every day.

Sometimes I was so tired, I was afraid of falling asleep while driving. I decided to ask for help driving to appointments.

CHAPTER 47
A NINETIES SITCOM

ON LABOR DAY weekend, smack-dab in the middle of radiation treatments, Jonathan's siblings, Zachary and Anna, moved to Utah from New York. Anna had planned to make the cross-country move before the pandemic, but COVID-19 delayed her plans.

A few weeks before Anna's scheduled move, Zachary decided he'd also like a change of scenery. He'd recently graduated from high school and was in a good place to make a fresh start. While Anna planned to get an apartment, Zachary asked if he could move in with us. Since we had converted my Reiki room and the entire second floor into a guest space, we agreed for him to move into the upstairs rooms where my mom had stayed a few months earlier.

Having an extra person in the house was nice, especially before Zachary settled into a work and school routine. Not only was it great to have additional help and company, but it was great to get to know him better. There's a seventeen-year age difference between Jonathan and Zachary, and Zach was just a baby when Jonathan moved out of their family home.

Having his brother around was good for Jonathan's spirit. There was laughter. There was reminiscing. There was storytelling. The joy radiating from Jonathan was something I hadn't seen for a long time. Seeing him genuinely smile and connect with his twenty-year-old brother made my heart happy.

Soon after our house turned into what felt like a nineties sitcom with people coming and going, Jonathan got word that he'd be going on a work trip to the East Coast. It would be his first post-pandemic work trip.

"Will you be OK if I go?" he asked. "I don't have to go if you're not cool with it."

"It'll be fine. Zach's here if I need anything." After I said that, I remembered my schedule for the next week. "Except . . . oh shoot."

"What's the matter?"

"I forgot that I have Kadcyla next week," I said. "So Kadcyla and radiation will be on the same day. And you'll be gone."

"Do you want to ask Zach if he can go with you? It might be good for him."

Until now, Jonathan was the only person to have seen me receive chemo. It felt like an intimate, personal thing. And even though Zachary lived with us now, he didn't know me very well.

Jonathan called his brother downstairs. "Zach, next week, I need to go on a work trip, and I'll be gone for just a few days."

"OK," The wheels were turning in Zachary's mind about what this meant for him.

"Emily will be here," Jonathan continued. "But she has an infusion and radiation on Tuesday. Would you be able to take her to those?"

Zachary's eyes brightened. He enjoyed helping others. "Sure, yeah, no problem," he agreed.

On Tuesday morning, Zachary and I left the house at seven o'clock, earlier than he was used to functioning. He drove slower than any twenty-year-old I knew. Maybe his beater of a car couldn't handle the hills, or maybe he was nervous about driving in a new place. I was worried we'd be late for radiation, but we made it on time.

"Do they have coffee around here?" he asked before I was called back.

"There's a Starbucks on the sixth floor," I said. "When you exit the elevator, go left and down the long hallway. You'll feel like you're going the wrong way, but keep going. It's back there, I promise." He nodded with a hesitant confidence and took off in pursuit of caffeine to make up for waking before the sun.

When I returned to the waiting room after my treatment, I saw Zachary holding a Starbucks cup in his hand.

"I just got back," he said. "I thought I was going the wrong way." The hospital had been under construction as long as I had been in treatment, and finding where to go wasn't always easy.

We got back in the car and headed an hour back to the infusion center for my nine thirty appointment. I was crossing my fingers that we'd make it in time. I felt stressed but tried to enjoy getting to know Zachary. I don't know what it is about young people in cars, but they tend to open up while driving. I felt sorry that we had lived so far away during his childhood and that this was the first time I was getting to know him.

When we got to the infusion center, we were led to a curtained-off infusion pod, just like always. Through getting my port accessed, blood drawn, and hooked up to the IV machine, I kept glancing at Zachary to make sure he was OK.

I was the healthiest-looking person there that day. I had a small amount of baby hair, and I could walk on my own. That constituted a healthy-looking person in the infusion center.

Others were bald as I had once been, in wheelchairs, or looked pale and unwell. Zachary's eyes were more alert than usual, and he sat on the edge of the visitor chair, looking at his phone.

"You OK?" I asked him.

"Yeah, yeah," he said, shifting in his seat. "I'm OK."

Even though he was an adult, I hoped that bringing him was a good choice. He called Karen when we got home to tell her about it.

"It's good for him," she said to Jonathan later. "Seeing people who have it tougher than us can have an impact on a young person. I'm glad he was there to help." I was, too.

I learned that sometimes people can handle more than we think they can, especially young people. I also learned that it was good for me to let others in—people besides Jonathan and my mom. People wanted to help. They were eager to help. I just had to let them.

CHAPTER 48

REAL-LIFE ANGELS

THE DAILY DRIVE to the hospital ate up a lot of time, but I found ways to look forward to it. I downloaded audiobooks from the local library and listened to them at double speed. I listened to eleven books over the six weeks. As my burns grew worse, my mind escaped into other worlds.

For the last day of radiation, I had written thank-you cards and included Starbucks gift cards for the entire radiation staff, including the receptionists who remembered my name every day. Now that I'm thinking about it, maybe the location tracker on my phone let them know I had arrived, but I like to think they remembered my name.

I walked into the radiation department with a skip in my step on that final day. Nothing made me happier than the thought of never going back there again.

I bounded into the women's waiting room for the last time, ready to tell everyone that it was *my* last day. But the room was empty. I was the only one there that morning. I felt ripped off. Who was I supposed to celebrate with?

My question was answered when I checked in at the name and birthday desk.

"Today's your last day!" Jennifer said. "I have something for you. I made it."

"You made something for me?" I asked as she handed me a piece of light blue fabric wrapped in white ribbon. I untied the ribbon and unfolded the fabric. It was a Soarin' T-shirt.

"I made it for your celebration trip to Disney," she said. Tears pooled in my eyes, and I hugged her. Her thoughtful gift made me realize how much I'd miss seeing my new friends every day.

"I'm going to wear it when I go," I said.

As I left the radiation treatment room for the final time, immense joy filled my entire being. The techs at the name and birthday desk handed me a completion certificate. I did a happy dance as I held it in my hand. To my surprise, Jennifer and every single person behind the desk started dancing with me. It was a group celebration.

At that moment, I was convinced that every person who worked at the cancer hospital was a real-life angel.

CHAPTER 49

WEDDING

FIVE DAYS AFTER finishing radiation, when the burns on my chest were at their worst, I got on a plane to Pennsylvania for my brother's wedding. I was in the middle of Kadcyla cycles and cleared to travel.

Because Jonathan was Jeffrey's best man, we dived headfirst into wedding duties: picking up tuxedos, helping with decorations, attending rehearsals, and most importantly, meeting my nephew for the first time. Jeffrey's son had been born during the pandemic, and between stay-at-home ordinances and getting cancer immediately afterward, I hadn't yet met my eighteen-month-old nephew.

Jonathan and I arrived at the bride's house to help her and her family finish putting together the decorations. I couldn't stand up for long due to the fatigue, so I sat on the front porch, which was filled with pumpkins to decorate the fall wedding. Unsure about this new, semi-bald lady who just showed up, my nephew took my sitting among the pumpkins as an invitation. One by one, he handed me each small pumpkin on the porch.

"Thank you," I said as he handed me another, and another, and another. I thanked him for each one and set each beside me. Sitting in a sea of teetering pumpkin piles, I realized that this was what I was fighting for. These were life's moments I didn't want to miss. I didn't care about fighting for myself. I had a good life. I was content. I was fighting to live for those around me. My family. My people.

I spent the rest of that day at Mom and Dad's house while Jonathan went out with the groomsmen for the bachelor party. My phone rang around dinnertime. It was Jonathan.

"Hey," he said. "Everyone wants to go to the indoor golf place, but I think we're going to be there late. Can your mom drive you back to the hotel?"

"Yeah, that's no problem," Mom said, overhearing the conversation. Her health had continued to improve since returning home from Utah.

"But I need to change out my bandage," I remembered. My radiation burns were at their worst, just days after the last treatment. "It's really gross."

"I can do it," Mom said. "It's OK."

After eating dinner, she drove me back to the hotel in town. I gathered the supplies needed to change the bandage and sat on the bed. Mom stood next to me, looking worried about what she was about to witness. She had seen straight into the hole in my chest, but she hadn't seen my burns yet.

I lifted my right arm and took it out of my shirt. Mom helped me gently remove my left arm from the sleeve.

"Are you ready?" I asked. "You don't have to help if you don't want to. It looks like Freddy Krueger."

"It's OK." She tried her best to be brave.

I released the Velcro closure from the Ace bandage and gingerly unwrapped it from my torso. I slowly removed the cut-up piece of T-shirt used to prevent the bandage from irritating my skin, or rather, the lack of skin. Two pieces of nonstick gauze remained. Unblinking, Mom was focused on what came next.

"I'm going to lift the gauze," I warned. "Don't pass out, OK?"

"I told you I'm OK," she insisted. But her words and body language didn't match.

I lifted the gauze, revealing bright red tissue that was oozing yellow. I was so inflamed that it looked like my incision was slit, running from the center of my chest into my armpit.

"My God, Emily." She sounded aghast. "How are you even here? You really shouldn't have traveled like this."

"It's important," I said. "I want to be here for big events. And if I'm able, then I'm going to."

Mom was my extra pair of hands as I re-dressed the wound. In order, I layered the burn cream, Aquaphor healing ointment, nonstick gauze, and a piece of T-shirt fabric. Then Mom helped me wind the Ace bandage around my body to secure everything in place. I found this surefire method from a fellow flattie's YouTube channel. You can learn anything from the internet.

The following day, Jonathan and I picked up his tuxedo and snacks for the groomsmen, and we headed to the Poconos for the wedding festivities.

I was excited to see my extended family that weekend. While in the depths of treatment, I had questioned whether I'd ever see my aunts, uncles, and cousins again. They always supported me from afar, but there was nothing like getting a big hug from my family.

"Emskee!" my uncle exclaimed as soon as he saw me from across the room. My immune system was still low, so I put on a sparkly pink face mask before receiving a giant bear hug. This was the reaction from each member of my family.

For the first time in a long time, I felt normal. I was out in the world participating in a normal life event. I wasn't in a doctor's office, an infusion center, or a hospital. I was in society among people who weren't part of a medical staff. I wasn't there as a sick person. I was there as the sister of the groom. I had done normal chores that morning, running errands and getting ready. It seemed so simple and mundane, yet it felt so significant. Being out in the real world was a surreal feeling, something I hadn't experienced in so long, yet there I was. I didn't know if I'd participate in these types of events ever again. I didn't know if I'd be around for them.

I might have had layers upon layers of bandages under my dress and been in pain every time I moved my arms, but I was there. I might have danced to the side of the dance floor to avoid being in a sea of people and their potential germs, but I was there. I might have had the thinnest of peach fuzz as hair, but I was there. I was doing a normal life thing with the people I love. I was there.

CHAPTER 50

THE REVOLVING DOOR AND RELATIONSHIPS

AS ACTIVE TREATMENT neared its end, I realized there was a significant evolution in many of my pre-cancer relationships. Some became stronger, some fizzled, and some became nonexistent. Having cancer led to a shift in how others perceived me and how I perceived others.

I saw this transition as a revolving door separating a beautiful, well-maintained building from the busy street outside. My old life was housed inside the building, sheltered and protected. Outside on the sidewalk, exposed to the elements, was my new life, my post-diagnosis life. Cancer had thrown me out onto the street and into the rain, snow, wind, and harsh rays of the sun. There was no going back inside. Those conditions would alter my body, soul, and mind forever. I would never unlearn what it meant to be affected by the harsh elements cancer brought my way. I would never be the way I was before. I'd be pelted, windswept, and beaten by this thing that happened to me.

Every person I knew before lived inside the building, in the pre-cancer world. Each would have the opportunity to step into and use the revolving door. As they rotated toward the outdoors, they would choose how they responded to the new version of me. They could step outside, supporting me through the challenge and accepting the changed version of me, or they could continue rotating and return to the familiarity of the building.

This option revealed three types of people. The first group would choose to keep going, spinning the door 360 degrees, and exiting on the same side from which they entered. They would ignore the new, changed version of me, pretending like I wasn't there. I call these people the avoiders. The second group would slow the door down as they approached the street and stick out their hand to wave, as if to say *Yeah, good luck with that!* But they would never stop. They would simply acknowledge me and continue the rotation to return inside. These are fair-weather friends. They're there when times are good and happy but can't be bothered when things get hard. The third group would jump out onto the street to support me, sometimes getting battered by cancer's elements in their own ways. These people stepped up and came through. These were my true friends, my close family, my people—my ride or dies.

What people chose to do while in the door allowed me to understand what their abilities were when it came to showing up for others. Some were not capable of being there for another person. They were going through their own struggles, their own battles. Others just didn't have it in them to make a sincere effort. Not everyone is cut out for something like this—watching a friend come close to death. It's easier for them to take a back seat and protect their heart in case the worst should happen. I understand why someone would do this, but I don't view those people as true friends.

It was disappointing to learn that some of my people were not capable of true friendship—that messy, raw friendship that isn't pretty but is authentic and meaningful. Several lifelong friends, people I was sure would jump into the street, ended up being avoiders. They never said a word to me during my entire cancer journey. These were people who, if in a similar situation, I would have flown to the other side of the world for and wiped their shitty ass if they needed me to. And yet when that revolving door passed me by, I knew the relationship was one-sided. I realize now that we were never walking out of that building together. The door would keep spinning and spinning. I could no longer keep these few people close.

Relationships are a two-way street. Healthy friendships require give-and-take from both people. When they're one-sided, there's an imbalance of effort and energy. I realized that I had experienced this with these friends. Withdrawing my energy from those relationships was painful. It stung. Especially when I was certain that these were my people. But they weren't. I had to accept that I was losing friends I once held dear.

The ride or dies showed up however I needed them to. These friendships were fueled by mutual love and support, where equal amounts of energy were exchanged. When one of us said, *Hey, I got you*, we meant it. And they did. These are the relationships that didn't change from when my pre-cancer self resided inside the protected building. These are the way things were, these are the way things are, and these are the way things should be. And that's a good feeling.

Losing avoiders and fair-weather friends created space for new relationships. They say the inflammatory breast cancer world is small, and I found that to be true. I met several IBC sisters on that imaginary street who were facing their own elements, their own challenges. That's where I met my IBC sister Sonja, who had a nearly identical diagnosis as I did. We walked through treatment side by side, comparing notes, leaning on each other for support through hard days, and cheering each other on through good days. This woman, once a stranger living states away, became one of my best friends for life. There is truth to the saying "It takes one to know one." When life's challenges bring people together in something very few can understand, an unbreakable bond is formed. In our case, a lifetime of sisterhood was born.

Cancer caused me to learn about people. I was made to create a sense of discernment within me about who people were at their core and what type of people I wanted, or didn't want, in my life moving forward. I am now more discerning in my relationships in a way I wasn't before. I sense someone's ability to nurture a two-way friendship nourished by equal effort. This is something I didn't anticipate needing to do before cancer entered my life. If I liked someone, they were my friend, and that was that. I have now found being choosy to be essential to positive emotional and mental health moving forward. We all have a limited amount of energy, including the energy we put into relationships, whether that be with friends, family, or romantic partners. For me, I choose to invest my energy in those who invest their energy in me. I choose to be friendly and cordial with everyone else, including avoiders and fair-weather friends, even if those people have decided that I am too different now to continue a relationship with.

Cancer is life-changing. None of us comes out the other side the same way we went in. There is no going back. It is normal for relationships to change in nature. And change is OK.

CHAPTER 51
MY "OLD SELF"

I BET YOU CAN'T WAIT to get back to your old self again.

If I had a dollar for every time someone said this to me, I could buy a nice meal at a fancy restaurant. But what happens when it's all said and done? What happens when you "beat" cancer, especially when it's rare, aggressive, and scary? Would I really go back to being my old self? Absolutely not.

Before I started treatment, I looked forward to putting cancer behind me. I wanted to fast-forward through the hard parts and return to life as I knew it. But I quickly learned that wasn't how it would go. My body was vastly different from what it had been just a year earlier, and the changes were apparent to anyone with eyeballs. My boobs were gone. I was weaker. My hair was thinner. I wasn't as vibrant as I had once been. The emotional, mental, and spiritual changes weren't as apparent to other people. They weren't outwardly visible, but I was very aware of their existence.

I had cancer. Nothing will ever be the same as it was before. I will never go back to being my old self. Everything is different now. The idea of going back to how things were seems great. I would love to not know the things I know now. I would love to be as naive and ignorant of suffering as I was before. But that's not how it is.

I've been through a kind of metaphorical fire. People often feel uncomfortable talking to people who have lost everything in a house fire. A common sentiment expressed to individuals who have lost all their belongings is *Thank God you got out OK.* Sure, they got out OK, but it doesn't mitigate the trauma of losing everything you once had. It's similar when it comes to cancer, but instead of losing my earthly possessions, I lost my breasts, my innocence, my relationships, my naivety, my eyebrows, my fertility, my worldview, and so much more. I look at the world completely differently now. I know things about human nature that I didn't know before. I know resilience. I know suffering. I know loss. I know what it is to look death in the face. Yet somehow, I'm supposed to forget that trauma, be grateful that I'm still alive, and "get back to my old self."

And I *am* grateful to be alive. Many times, when someone asks how I'm doing, I reply, "Just happy to be here." And I mean it. Through the fire, I've learned about life and how precious it is. I sometimes get frustrated when I perceive that others might not understand these same things.

Soon after finishing chemo, I went to the grocery store to shop for the first time in a year. It was like being teleported to another place and time. It felt surreal. People bustled around with their shopping carts, checking the freshness of produce and expiration dates on boxes and jars. I felt like I was outside of myself, watching the world happen from a third-party perspective. I wondered if any of those people appreciated their health, or if they were simply going along with the expected motions of everyday life. I wanted to shout, *Do you guys know how precious life is?* Before cancer, I too went through life, checking produce without a care in the world. I didn't grasp how amazing it was to be alive. I didn't appreciate it the way I do now.

However, being grateful to be alive doesn't soften the effect of all the ways cancer has changed me. The feeling of euphoria that follows the end of treatment eventually fades. Real life creeps back in. While my world came to a halt during treatment, the world began to spin again once the poison left my body, and I slowly regained my strength. When Zachary went away to college, I set up my Reiki studio and began seeing clients again. But the unexpected happened. Doing Reiki didn't feel the same as when I had left it. Even though I was more hopeful for the future than ever before, I had changed. My dreams had changed. So I paused my Reiki practice again and will go back to it when it feels right.

My life appeared to be returning to normal. My hair started growing back, but not in the way I thought it would. Most people are blessed with thick, curly hair following chemotherapy. I was looking forward to that and bought cute hair accessories to adorn my new chemo curls. However, that's not what happened. My hair came in thin, fine, and poker straight. I was disappointed, but I told everyone I was just happy to have my hair back. My skin regained its color, pinkening up and losing its pale, yellowish hue. I joined a doctor-led fitness program at the hospital and slowly built muscle and gained endurance. I no longer needed a cane to walk. The outward signs of my illness were disappearing one by one, and I appeared more "normal." I looked different than my pre-cancer self, but not sickly.

Some friends' presence evaporated along with the signs that I was a cancer patient. As I appeared less sickly and rejoined society, people assumed I was good. I was anything but good. Maybe they were burnt out from always hearing about cancer or being around a sick person. Maybe they became busy with their own lives and families. I can't pretend to know the reason, and I don't fault anyone for this. The world doesn't revolve around me. But life after cancer is lonely. It's maddening.

Fear of cancer recurrence and hypothetical thoughts consumed my mind in the years after treatment. *What if the cancer comes back? What if I never regain my full strength? What if I can never work a "real" job again because of chemo brain? What if I beat cancer only to die in some freak accident one day?* Logically, I know there's nothing I can do to control these things. I can only do what I can to live as healthily as I can—get checkups, eat nutritious foods, exercise regularly, and do my best to reduce stress. It's hard to reduce stress when I'm in constant fear of the cancer returning, but I do my best. I meditate, I participate in activities that bring me joy, and I surround myself with people I love. I also make a conscious effort to reject the opposite of those things. I no longer accept anything other than love and kindness from others. I do my best to turn those anxious thoughts around and into affirmations. *I beat cancer. I beat the statistics. I have a beautiful life. I live in a beautiful place. I'm surrounded by incredible people.* Those thoughts get me through each day and fill my heart with hope.

I gave up trying to find the meaning in every detail of what happened to me. Not every shift is a loss, and not every loss is a lesson. Sometimes it's just a loss. Sometimes things just happen. And that's OK. I found that trying to find meaning in every minute detail of my experience was a form of toxic positivity. For me, it was best to let my experience simply be my experience. It happened, and it was what it was.

I had to find a way to move on, to move forward. I embraced the parts of me that hadn't changed—my feisty personality, my weird sense of humor, my love of harmless pranks and jokes. I embraced my femininity, even without breasts. They don't define me as a woman anyway. I am more than boobs. I embraced the values and morals I hold and began outwardly standing up for what I believe is true and right. I embraced opportunities to be present for others. I embraced love and kindness in my daily life. After all, I'm still me at my core. I'm the same weirdo who loves deep dives into genealogy research, Taylor Swift, true crime documentaries, and planning Halloween costumes four months in advance. I still can't carry a tune to save my life, and I still sing in the car as if I can. I'm still me. I'm still Emily. She made it through the fire.

Although I do my best to stay optimistic and quash invasive thoughts when they creep up, I'm not naive about IBC recurrence rates. According to a study on the patterns of recurrence performed at M.D. Anderson Cancer Center, within five years of diagnosis, 64.8 percent of IBC patients will experience a cancer recurrence. That's almost two-thirds of us. That's a lot. Funding and research can change that. Organizations like the Inflammatory Breast Cancer Research Foundation, The IBC Network Foundation, and the American Cancer Society have dedicated hundreds of thousands of dollars toward research and treatment advancements. Improvements are made to the IBC treatment protocol with each medical trial, giving us a chance at a better prognosis. Cancer research is being done every day, always moving forward. There is always hope.

CHAPTER 52
THE END?

WALKING INTO THE infusion center for the last time was surreal. While arriving always made me anxious because I knew I'd feel like garbage for the next few weeks, this place had also become a second home. I spent a lot of time there. It was a place of healing, where I was pumped full of the substance that would ultimately save my life. I got to know the nurses, and they got to know me. It was strange knowing this was the last time I'd be here with these people doing this thing. This was the end of active treatment.

As fate would have it, I was assigned to the exact chair where I received my first chemotherapy infusion just over a year earlier. The universe brought me full circle. I didn't read, play games, or listen to music during this final session. I reclined the chair and closed my eyes to reflect on the woman sitting there now versus the woman who sat there a year ago.

Everything is different now. This thing, this cancer, this experience, shook me to my core. But it turned out that my core was unshakable. I'm going to be OK. That wasn't something I believed going in, but I know it coming out.

Going in, I didn't know if I'd come out alive, let alone alive and functional. Forget about being functional and in a good mental place. But here I am. My core hung on, and this is how I go forward.

My past self, the me who was sobbing in a fetal position on the living room floor, convinced she couldn't go on, the me I wrote this book for, would have wanted to know if it was all worth it. Did she turn out OK? How did it end? I'm proud to tell her that she's stronger, braver, and more resilient than she ever imagined. She accomplished great things and can hold her head high. But there is no ending to this.

An ending doesn't happen here because I got to live. This will be with me in some way or another forever. My soul has changed. The person I am is forever changed. I'll go for six-month checkups for the rest of my life. I'll continue to take medication, keeping any unknown rogue cancer cells at bay, for years to come. This doesn't go away like a bad dream. For some people with different illnesses, they recover, and it all becomes a distant memory. That's not how it is for me, or anyone with IBC. It continues on. And on and on. Every time I look down at my chest and see my scars, I'm reminded of this thing that happened. I'm not moving on from it, I'm moving on with it.

The IV pump beeped for the last time, and the nurse detached the machine from my port. I was free. Jonathan gathered my blanket and bags. I became misty-eyed as I picked up my tote.

"We have some things for you since this is your last day," the nurse said, handing me a bright yellow piece of paper, a completion certificate signed by all the staff. Then she gave me a blanket. Just what I needed!

"Are you going to ring the bell?" she asked.

"Heck yeah!" I beamed. She parted the curtain and led us down the hallway. A bell hung on the wall just before the exit. One of the nurses took my phone and started recording.

"Ring it hard," another nurse said from the background.

Clutching my coat and my twelfth gifted blanket with one arm, I grabbed the bell's cord and rang it as hard as I could for all to hear. Everyone in the place would know that I just accomplished the hardest thing I would ever do. I jumped up and down and threw my fist into the air. I felt like a champion. An exhausted, beat-up, accomplished champion.

"That's the hardest anyone has ever rung the bell," my nurse said. "Usually people just ring it once or twice, but you really went for it."

"I've been looking forward to that for so long," I said. It was just a bell on a wall, but it symbolized so much. It was resilience. It was perseverance. It was accomplishment. It was life. It was also recognition that not everyone would ring this bell. Some would never make it to the bell. For those friends who would always remain in my heart, it symbolized honor, respect, and remembrance.

"Can I give you a hug before you go?" she asked. "I'm so happy for you, but I'll miss you."

"I'll miss you, too." I gave her a long, tight embrace.

I walked out of the infusion center for the last time and into a warm spring afternoon. I was officially moving on to the next phase of life. I didn't know what that looked like yet. I didn't have a plan. I didn't know much for sure. The only thing I knew was that IBC would not crush my spirit. I would not break from this. Not from this.

Scan the QR code for a video of Emily ringing the bell and photos from throughout her treatment journey, many of which are mentioned throughout this book.

HELPFUL RECIPES

PLEASE CONSULT your health-care provider before using any products on your body to ensure their safety for your specific situation.

Scalp Shampoo
Mix vitamin E oil and essential oils into the shampoo bottle. I used a wooden skewer to mix it together. Every other day, wash your scalp just as you would your hair to remove excess oils and keep your skin clean.
- 500mL calendula shampoo
- 1 tsp vitamin E oil
- 33 drops rosemary essential oil
- 33 drops lemon essential oil

Scalp Oil
After bathing, use a cotton round or cotton cloth to distribute oil on your clean scalp.
- 1½ oz jojoba oil
- 1½ oz grapeseed oil
- 30 drops clary sage essential oil
- 30 drops cedarwood essential oil
- 30 drops rosemary essential oil

Mouth Rinse
This recipe was provided by my oncology nurse for mouth sores and mouth burning. I found it to be very effective. Rinse with this several times per day. (I rinsed every time I used the bathroom.) Make a new batch each day to ensure freshness. I'm not sure the size of the Mason jar matters, but this is what I did.

In a quart-size Mason jar, mix together:
1 tsp salt
1 tsp baking soda
Fill the rest with water.

Radiation Chest Wrap
I modified this technique learned from a fellow flattie. Re-dress your chest twice a day, every morning and evening.

Layer in this order:
Prescription burn cream
Aquaphor ointment (from the tub, not tube, as it takes less physical strength to scoop out)
Nonstick gauze
T-shirt material
Wrap torso with a 6-inch-wide Ace bandage (with Velcro closure).

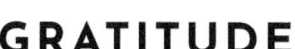

GRATITUDE

To my Mama: It's you and me forever. Thank you for teaching me how to be strong, kind, and braver than a bee. I'm forever grateful to inherit this feisty personality and incredible resilience. Cosma would be proud.

To Jonathan: Thank you for always loving, supporting, and encouraging me in sickness and in health. I will always appreciate your unwavering belief in me. Your humor and wonderfully strange sayings remind me that dark days can still hold laughter and hope. I love you beyond measure!

To my family: Thank you for showing up in all the ways that matter most. Your patience, sense of humor, and unconditional love are what get me through every challenge. I love you mucho!

To my friends: Thank you for all your support and love. I cherish each of you beyond words.

To my IBC and flattie sisters: You are each a constant inspiration to me. Your strength, perseverance, and beauty are everything. Here's to living life every day! YODO!

To Cindy Childress, my incredible writing coach and fairy godmother: Thank you for lighting a fire under my butt to make this book a reality. Your guidance and support along the way have been immeasurable.

To my editing, design, and publishing team at The Writer's Ally—Ally Machate, Julie Haase, Hannah Diedrich, Michele Rubin, Emily King, Emily Hitchcock, Clair Fink, Amy Handy: Thank you for helping me turn my vision into a reality. You're all incredibly talented and magical! A special thank you to my editors, Michele Rubin and Emily King. To Michele: It felt like you took a trip into my mind, saw my vision, and helped me find the words to express it. Thank you for your honesty, your patience, and your talent! To Emily: Your care and precision brought heart to every detail of my story. Thank you for treating my words with such kindness and skill! You are truly amazing.

To every doctor, surgeon, nurse, radiation tech, physical therapist, social worker, receptionist, maintenance staff member, security guard, and everyone else at Huntsman Cancer Institute: Thank you for saving lives every day. You are angels on Earth, and you're loved beyond measure. I would quite literally not be here without you. Thank you.

To Dr. B: Thank you for your incredible kindness and empathy. Your presence was the calm through the IBC storm. Your unwavering belief that healing was possible and your expertise gave me a future I wasn't sure I'd have. I'm forever grateful. My next plant will be named in your honor.

Hope always!

If you're able, please consider donating to the following organizations. Funding for continued research and outreach saves lives. Your help is desperately needed and greatly appreciated.

Inflammatory Breast Cancer Research Foundation
ibcresearch.org/get-involved/donate

The IBC Network Foundation
theibcnetwork.org/donate

American Cancer Society
cancer.org/donate

BIBLIOGRAPHY

American Cancer Society. "Inflammatory Breast Cancer." 2025. https://www.cancer.org/cancer/types/breast-cancer/about/types-of-breast-cancer/inflammatory-breast-cancer.html.

Cancer Council. "Studies Say Dogs Could Be Trained to Sniff Out Cancer." Updated January 2024. https://www.cancer.org.au/iheard/can-animals-sniff-out-cancer.

Chang, Edward I., Roman J. Skoracki, and David W. Chang. "Lymphovenous Anastomosis Bypass Surgery." *Seminars in Plastic Surgery* 32 , no. 1 (2018): 22–27. https://doi.org/10.1055/s-0038-1636510. Retrieved from https://pmc.ncbi.nlm.nih.gov/articles/PMC5891648/.

Cristofanilli, Massimo, Vicente Valero, Aman U. Buzdar, et al. (2007). "Inflammatory Breast Cancer (IBC) and Patterns of Recurrence." *Cancer* 110, no. 7 (2007): 1436–1444. https://doi.org/10.1002/cncr.22927.

Dana-Farber Cancer Institute. "Deep Inspiration Breath-Hold Technique." 2025. https://www.dana-farber.org/health-library/videos/

radiation-therapy-for-breast-cancer-deep-inspiration-breath-hold#.

Nicaise, Benjamin, Pierre Loap, Delphine Loirat, et al. "Radiotherapy in the Management of Non-Metastatic Inflammatory Breast Cancers: A Retrospective Observational Study." *Cancers* 14, no. 1 (2021): 107. https://doi.org/10.3390/cancers14010107. Retrieved from https://pmc.ncbi.nlm.nih.gov/articles/PMC8750160/.

Ross, Tracee E. "Tracee Ellis Ross Speaks up for Childless Women at Kamala Harris' Event." AssociatedPress. September 20, 2024. Video, 0:00:15, https://www.youtube.com/shorts/ClnLHe6xaj0.

U.S. Department of Health and Human Services, National Institutes of Health, National Cancer Institute. "Inflammatory Breast Cancer." Reviewed January 2016. https://www.cancer.gov/types/breast/ibc-fact-sheet.

von Minckwitz, Gunter, Chiun-Sheng Huang, Max S. Mano, et al. "Trastuzumab Emtansine for Residual Invasive HER2-Positive Breast Cancer." *The New England Journal of Medicine* 380, no. 7 (2018): 617–628. https://doi.org/10.1056/NEJMoa1814017.

ABOUT THE AUTHOR

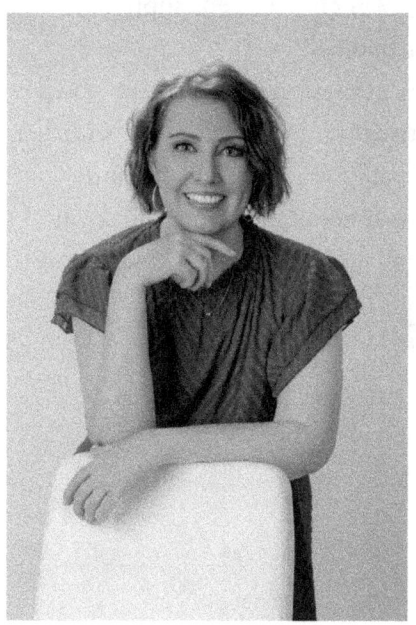

EMILY JUNGBLUT is a breast cancer survivor, writer, and communications professional passionate about using storytelling to inspire hope and advocacy. After being diagnosed with inflammatory breast cancer at thirty-five, she made it her mission to talk about what most people whisper — to normalize conversations about boobs, bodies, and the messy parts of healing nobody talks about.

Through her writing, speaking, and digital platforms, Emily advocates for early detection, emotional resilience, and the power of humor through hard times. She blends personal experience with her professional background to show that vulnerability can be both a form of education and empowerment. Emily's goal is simple: to help women feel seen, supported, and unashamed to talk about their bodies.

When she's not writing or studying, you'll probably find her hiking, cross-stitching, or hanging out with her family, friends, and cats—preferably with a coffee in hand.

Connect with her at emilyjungblut.com.

www.ingramcontent.com/pod-product-compliance
Lightning Source LLC
Chambersburg PA
CBHW020536030426
42337CB00013B/878